Pediatric Infectious Disease: Part II

Editors

MARY ANNE JACKSON
ANGELA L. MYERS

INFECTIOUS DISEASE CLINICS
OF NORTH AMERICA

www.id.theclinics.com

Consulting Editor
HELEN W. BOUCHER

December 2015 • Volume 29 • Number 4

ELSEVIER

1600 John F. Kennedy Boulevard • Suite 1800 • Philadelphia, Pennsylvania, 19103-2899.
http://www.theclinics.com

INFECTIOUS DISEASE CLINICS OF NORTH AMERICA Volume 29, Number 4
December 2015 ISSN 0891-5520, ISBN-13: 978-0-323-40252-1

Editor: Kerry Holland
Developmental Editor: Donald Mumford

Infectious Disease Clinics of North America (ISSN 0891-5520) is published in March, June, September, and December by Elsevier Inc., 360 Park Avenue South, New York, NY 10010-1710. Periodicals postage paid at New York, NY and additional mailing offices. Subscription prices are $295.00 per year for US individuals, $510.00 per year for US institutions, $145.00 per year for US students, $350.00 per year for Canadian individuals, $638.00 per year for Canadian institutions, $420.00 per year for international individuals, $638.00 per year for international institutions, and $200.00 per year for Canadian and international students. To receive student rate, orders must be accompanied by name of affiliated institution, date of term, and the *signature* of program/residency coordinator on institution letterhead. Orders will be billed at individual rate until proof of status is received. Foreign air speed delivery is included in all *Clinics* subscription prices. All prices are subject to change without notice. **POSTMASTER:** Send address changes to *Infectious Disease Clinics of North America*, Elsevier Health Sciences Division, Subcription Customer Service, 3251 Riverport Lane, Maryland Heights, MO 63043. **Customer Service: 1-800-654-2452 (US). From outside of the US and Canada, call 1-314-447-8871. Fax: 1-314-447-8029. E-mail: JournalsCustomerService-usa@elsevier.com (print support) or JournalsOnlineSupport-usa@elsevier.com (online support).**

Infectious Disease Clinics of North America is also published in Spanish by Editorial Inter-Médica, Junin 917, 1er A 1113, Buenos Aires, Argentina.

Reprints. For copies of 100 or more, of articles in this publication, please contact the Commercial Reprints Department, Elsevier Inc., 360 Park Avenue South, New York, New York 10010-1710. Tel. 212-633-3874, Fax: 212-633-3820, E-mail: reprints@elsevier.com.

Infectious Disease Clinics of North America is covered in *MEDLINE/PubMed (Index Medicus), Current Contents/Clinical Medicine, Science Citation Alert, SCISEARCH,* and *Research Alert.*

Contributors

CONSULTING EDITOR

HELEN W. BOUCHER, MD, FIDSA, FACP
Director, Infectious Diseases Fellowship Program, Division of Geographic Medicine and Infectious Diseases, Tufts Medical Center; Associate Professor of Medicine, Tufts University School of Medicine, Boston, Massachusetts

EDITORS

MARY ANNE JACKSON, MD, FAAP, FPIDS, FIDSA
Division of Pediatric Infectious Diseases, Director of Pediatric Infectious Diseases and Associate Chair of Pediatrics, Children's Mercy Hospital; Professor of Pediatrics, University of Missouri-Kansas City School of Medicine, Kansas City, Missouri

ANGELA L. MYERS, MD, MPH, FAAP, FPIDS
Division of Pediatric Infectious Diseases, Director, Travel Medicine; Director, Pediatric Infectious Diseases Fellowship Training Program, Children's Mercy Hospitals and Clinics; Associate Professor of Pediatrics, University of Missouri-Kansas City School of Medicine, Kansas City, Missouri

AUTHORS

KEVIN A. AULT, MD
Professor and Division Director, Department of Obstetrics and Gynecology, University of Kansas Medical Center, Kansas City, Kansas

HENRY H. BERNSTEIN, DO, MHCM
Professor of Pediatrics, Department of Pediatrics, Cohen Children's Medical Center of NY, Hofstra Northshore-LIJ School of Medicine, New Hyde Park, New York

JOHN C. CHRISTENSON, MD
Director, Pediatric Travel Medicine, Professor of Clinical Pediatrics, Chief, Clinical Services, Ryan White Center for Pediatric Infectious Disease and Global Health, Indiana University School of Medicine, Riley Hospital for Children at IU Health, Indianapolis, Indiana

STEPHEN L. COCHI, MD, MPH
Senior Advisor, Global Immunization Division, Center for Global Health Centers for Disease Control and Prevention, Atlanta, Georgia

AMANDA COHN, MD
Immunization Services Division, National Center for Immunization and Respiratory Diseases, Centers for Disease Control and Prevention, Atlanta, Georgia

PENELOPE H. DENNEHY, MD
Division of Pediatric Infectious Diseases, Department of Pediatrics, Hasbro Children's Hospital, Professor of Pediatrics, The Alpert Medical School of Brown University, Providence, Rhode Island

JULIE R. GARON, MPH
Manager, Research Projects, Division of Infectious Diseases, Emory University School of Medicine, Atlanta, Georgia

JAMES L. GOODSON, BSN, MPH
Global Immunization Division, Center for Global Health, Centers for Disease Control and Prevention, Atlanta, Georgia

ROBYN A. LIVINGSTON, MD
Associate Professor of Pediatrics, Division of Infectious Diseases, Department of Pediatrics, Children's Mercy Kansas City; University of Missouri-Kansas City School of Medicine, Kansas City, Missouri

SARAH S. LONG, MD
Professor, Section of Infectious Diseases, Department of Pediatrics, St. Christopher's Hospital for Children, Drexel University College of Medicine, Philadelphia, Pennsylvania

JESSICA MACNEIL, MPH
Bacterial Diseases Division, National Center for Immunization and Respiratory Diseases, Centers for Disease Control and Prevention, Atlanta, Georgia

ANGELA L. MYERS, MD, MPH, FAAP, FPIDS
Division of Pediatric Infectious Diseases, Director, Travel Medicine; Director, Pediatric Infectious Diseases Fellowship Training Program, Children's Mercy Hospitals and Clinics; Associate Professor of Pediatrics, University of Missouri-Kansas City School of Medicine, Kansas City, Missouri

WALTER A. ORENSTEIN, MD, DSc(Hon)
Associate Director, Emory Vaccine Center, Emory University School of Medicine, Atlanta, Georgia

BARBARA A. PAHUD, MD, MPH
Assistant Professor of Pediatrics, Division of Infectious Diseases, Department of Pediatrics, Children's Mercy Hospital, University of Missouri, Kansas City (UMKC), Kansas City, Missouri

STEPHEN I. PELTON, MD
Professor of Pediatrics and Epidemiology, Section of Pediatric Infectious Diseases, Department of Pediatrics, Maxwell Finland Laboratory for Infectious Diseases, Boston University Medical Center; Department of Epidemiology, Boston University School of Public Health, Boston, Massachusetts

JANE F. SEWARD, MBBS, MPH
Division of Viral Diseases, National Center for Immunization and Respiratory Diseases, Centers for Disease Control and Prevention, Atlanta, Georgia

KIMBERLY M. SHEA, PhD, MPH
Assistant Professor of Epidemiology, Department of Epidemiology, Boston University School of Public Health, Boston, Massachusetts

MICHAEL J. SMITH, MD, MSCE
Associate Professor of Pediatrics, Division of Pediatric Infectious Diseases, University of Louisville School of Medicine, Louisville, Kentucky

EMILY SOUDER, MD
Clinical Instructor, Section of Infectious Diseases, Department of Pediatrics, St. Christopher's Hospital for Children, Drexel University College of Medicine, Philadelphia, Pennsylvania

RODNEY E. WILLOUGHBY Jr, MD
Professor, Pediatrics (Infectious Diseases), Medical College of Wisconsin; Attending Physician, Pediatric Infectious Diseases, Children's Hospital of Wisconsin, Milwaukee, Wisconsin

INCI YILDIRIM, MD, MSc
Assistant Professor of Pediatrics, Section of Pediatric Infectious Diseases, Department of Pediatrics, Maxwell Finland Laboratory for Infectious Diseases, Boston University Medical Center; Department of Epidemiology, Boston University School of Public Health, Boston, Massachusetts

Contents

Influenza infects 5% to 20% of school-age children annually. Although universal influenza vaccine is recommended for children and adults 6 months of age and older, uptake is below national targets. Influenza immunization of the child and the family is the key to decreasing annual disease burden. Antiviral therapy is an important treatment strategy for children and adults, especially those who are at high risk of complications from influenza, irrespective of immunization status or whether illness onset is greater than 48 hours. Although antiviral therapy may also be used for pre-exposure and postexposure prophylaxis, it should not replace immunization as a preventive strategy when immunization is feasible.

Rotavirus infection is the most common cause of severe diarrhea disease in infants and young children worldwide. Vaccination is the only control measure likely to have a significant impact on the incidence of severe disease. Rotavirus vaccines have reduced the burden of disease in the United States and Europe and vaccine programs are being introduced in Asia and Africa where it is hoped that vaccine will have significant impact on severe infection. Long-term monitoring and strain surveillance are needed to assess the effects of rotavirus immunization programs and to determine whether changes in strain ecology will affect rotavirus vaccine effectiveness.

Rabies is an acute, rapidly progressive encephalitis that is almost always fatal. Prophylaxis is highly effective but economics limits disease control. The mechanism of death from rabies is unclear. It is poorly cytopathic and poorly inflammatory. Rabies behaves like an acquired metabolic disorder. There may be a continuum of disease severity. History of animal bite is rare. The diagnosis is often missed. Intermittent encephalopathy, dysphagia, hydrophobia and aerophobia, and focal paresthesias or myoclonic jerks suggest rabies. Laboratory diagnosis is cumbersome but sensitive. Treatment is controversial but survivors are increasingly reported, with good outcomes in 4 of 8 survivors.

In the United States during the 1950's, polio was on the forefront of every provider and caregiver's mind. Today, most providers in the United States have never seen a case. The Global Polio Eradication Initiative (GPEI), which began in 1988 has reduced the number of cases by over 99%. The world is closer to achieving global eradication of polio than ever before but as long as poliovirus circulates anywhere in the world, every country is vulnerable. The global community can support the polio eradication effort through continued vaccination, surveillance, enforcing travel regulations and contributing financial support, partnerships and advocacy.

The incidence of meningococcal disease is at an historic low in the United States, but prevention remains a priority because of the devastating outcomes and risk for outbreaks. Available vaccines are recommended routinely for persons at increased risk for disease to protect against all major serogroups of Neisseria meningitidis circulating in the United States. Although vaccination has virtually eliminated serogroup A meningococcal outbreaks from the Meningitis Belt of Africa and reduced the incidence of serogroup C disease worldwide, eradication of N meningitidis will unlikely be achieved by currently available vaccines because of the continued carriage and transmission of nonencapsulated organisms.

Universal immunization of infants and toddlers with pneumococcal conjugate vaccines over the last 15 years has dramatically altered the landscape of pneumococcal disease. Decreases in invasive pneumococcal disease, all-cause pneumonia, empyema, mastoiditis, acute otitis media, and complicated otitis media have been reported from multiple countries in which universal immunization has been implemented. Children with comorbid conditions have higher rates of pneumococcal disease and increased case fatality rates compared with otherwise healthy children, and protection for the most vulnerable pediatric patients will require new strategies to address the underlying host susceptibility and the expanded spectrum of serotypes observed.

Despite implementation of a successful vaccination program, pertussis remains a significant health problem. Although the incidence of pertussis in the United States is reduced by approximately 80% compared with incidence before the introduction of vaccination in the 1940s, deaths still occur and the unrecognized disease burden remains high, with 1 million Bordetella pertussis infections annually in the United States estimated by serologic surveys. Reasons for the resurgence and current prevalence of pertussis may be multifactorial and include waning vaccine-induced protection as well as lower vaccine effectiveness, failure to vaccinate, and changes in the organism itself.

Human papilloma virus (HPV) infection is the most common sexually transmitted infection in the United States. Some infections will result in anogenital warts and anogenital or oropharyngeal cancers. Preventing HPV infection is a public health priority to reduce cancer and HPV-associated complications. Prevention through vaccination is the most cost-effective and lifesaving intervention to decrease the burden of HPV-related cancers and other HPV-associated diseases. It is critical for pediatricians to make a strong recommendation for early and timely vaccination and completion of the 3-dose series. The goal of early vaccination is to immunize before first exposure to HPV virus.

In response to severe measles, the first measles vaccine was licensed in the United States in 1963. Widespread use of measles vaccines for more than 50 years has significantly reduced global measles morbidity and mortality. However, measles virus continues to circulate, causing infection, illness, and an estimated 400 deaths worldwide each day. Measles is preventable by vaccine, and humans are the only reservoir. Clinicians should promote and provide on-time vaccination for all patients and keep measles in their differential diagnosis of febrile rash illness for rapid case detection, confirmation of measles infection, isolation, treatment, and appropriate public health response.

Children are traveling to regions of the world that could pose a risk of acquiring diseases such as malaria, dermatosis, and infectious diarrhea. Most of these can be prevented by modifying high-risk behaviors or through the use of medications. Many of these same regions are endemic with diseases that are preventable through vaccination. Clinicians must be able to effectively prepare their pediatric-age travelers for international travel. Preventive education, prophylactic and self-treating medications, and vaccinations are all important components of this preparation. Familiarity with the use of travel vaccines is imperative.

Vaccine hesitancy incorporates a wide range of parental attitudes and behaviors surrounding vaccines. Ironically, the very success of the immunization program has fueled vaccine concerns; because vaccine-preventable diseases are no longer prevalent, attention has shifted to the safety and necessity of vaccines themselves. This article reviews some of the underlying themes of vaccine hesitancy as well as specific vaccine safety concerns. Strategies for discussing vaccines with concerned parents are also discussed.

INFECTIOUS DISEASE CLINICS OF NORTH AMERICA

FORTHCOMING ISSUES

March 2016
Fungal Infections
Luis Z. Ostrosky and Jack Sobel, *Editors*

June 2016
Antibiotic Resistance
Robert A. Bonomo and
Richard R. Watkins, *Editors*

September 2016
**Infection Prevention and Control in
Healthcare, Part I: Facility Planning
and Management**
Keith S. Kaye, *Editor*

RECENT ISSUES

September 2015
Pediatric Infectious Disease: Part I
Mary Anne Jackson and Angela L. Myers,
Editors

June 2015
**Lyme Disease and Other Infections
Transmitted by *Ixodes scapularis***
Paul G. Auwaeter, *Editor*

March 2015
Clostridium difficile Infection
Mark H. Wilcox, *Editor*

INFECTIOUS DISEASE CLINICS
OF NORTH AMERICA

Preface

Pediatric Infectious Diseases, Part 2

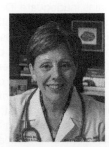
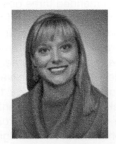

Mary Anne Jackson, MD, FAAP, FPIDS, FIDSA   Angela L. Myers, MD, MPH, FAAP, FPIDS
Editors

We are delighted to present this second issue of *Infectious Disease Clinics of North America* devoted to pediatrics and featuring state-of-the-art reviews related to pediatric vaccine-preventable infections.

We are proud to have enlisted authors who are exceptional national and international leaders and key subject matter experts in the field of communicable disease and childhood immunizations. We feel this issue offers comprehensive, state-of-the-art summaries focused on some of the most important advances and challenges related to pediatric immunization. Diseases and vaccines covered include influenza, rotavirus, rabies, poliomyelitis, meningococcus, pneumococcus, pertussis, human papillomavirus, measles, and travel-related vaccines.

The topic of influenza is covered by Drs Bernstein and Livingston, who outline the clinical manifestations, morbidity, and mortality of pediatric infection and the success and challenges related to influenza vaccination. Dr Dennehy highlights the success of the national rotavirus vaccine program and the remarkable impact on the incidence of rotavirus disease, describing rotavirus enteritis in young infants as possibly a disease of the past. Dr Rodney Willoughby provides an inclusive discussion of rabies disease, diagnosis and treatment, and outlines the approach to pre-exposure and postexposure prophylaxis. Drs Orenstein, Cochi, and Julie Garon elegantly describe the prospects of global elimination of poliomyelitis, focusing on the role that US physicians play in surveillance, vaccination, advocacy, and support of the global initiative for polio eradication. Drs Cohn and Jessica McNeil note that meningococcal disease is at an all-time low and outline the recommendations for the currently available meningo coccal vaccines, including the new meningococcal B vaccines. Drs Pelton, Yildirim, and Kimberly Shea highlight the dramatic change in the epidemiology of pneumococcal infection in the era of conjugate vaccines over the last 15 years and spotlight the role for new strategies to address the disproportionate burden of pneumococcal infection, which occurs in children with underlying host susceptibilities. The topic of

Infect Dis Clin N Am 29 (2015) xiii–xiv
http://dx.doi.org/10.1016/j.idc.2015.09.001
0891-5520/15/$ – see front matter © 2015 Published by Elsevier Inc.

id.theclinics.com

pertussis is covered by Drs Long and Souder, who provide a state-of-the-art discussion of the diagnosis and management, and the barriers to eradication, owing to changes in the organism and potential limitation of the currently available acellular pertussis vaccines. Drs Pahud and Ault discuss the spectrum of HPV-associated cancers and the role for and success thus far of the US HPV vaccine program, noting that despite ongoing efforts from providers and established guidelines, national coverage with the recommended three doses of HPV vaccine remains inadequate. Drs Seward and Goodson present a state-of-the-art review on measles, with a description of the current outbreak status in the United States related to importation of cases, emphasizing that practitioners must remain vigilant to maintain measles outbreak preparedness and the rapid response necessary to contain outbreaks. Drs Christenson and Myers provide a comprehensive vaccination approach to the traveling child with discussion of vaccine efficacy for specific diseases, and up-to-date information regarding risks of vaccine-preventable diseases in developing nations. Last, Dr Smith provides an overview of the problem of vaccine hesitancy, emphasizing the most effective communication strategies for effective vaccine risk communication that should be utilized with parents.

We hope that pediatric providers, including infectious diseases physicians and others, find this volume helpful to their practice. We would like to thank all of the authors for their contributions, and we especially recognize Jane Seward, who completed her work while deployed in Sierra Leone, Africa, where she was initiating a CDC-sponsored Ebola vaccine study. We again thank the editors, especially Donald Mumford, for helping us keep the issue on track, and Dr Helen Boucher, for inviting us to compile this issue. It has truly been a labor of love for us to bring this issue to you.

Mary Anne Jackson, MD, FAAP, FPIDS, FIDSA
Infectious Diseases
Children's Mercy Hospital
University of Missouri-
Kansas City School of Medicine
2401 Gillham Road
Kansas City, MO 64108, USA

Angela L. Myers, MD, MPH, FAAP, FPIDS
Children's Mercy Hospital
University of Missouri-
Kansas City School of Medicine
2401 Gillham Road
Kansas City, MO 64108, USA

E-mail addresses:
mjackson@cmh.edu (M.A. Jackson)
amyers@cmh.edu (A.L. Myers)

Prevention of Influenza in Children

Robyn A. Livingston, MD[a,b],*, Henry H. Bernstein, DO, MHCM[c]

KEYWORDS

- Influenza • Vaccine • Antivirals • Treatment • Chemoprophylaxis

KEY POINTS

- Vaccination remains the best available preventive measure against influenza.
- Annual seasonal influenza vaccine is recommended for all people 6 months and older, including children and adolescents.
- Vaccine effectiveness can vary based on the match or mismatch of circulating viruses with vaccine strains, vaccine product, and age and immune state of patients.
- Antiviral medications are important in the control of influenza, but are not a substitute for influenza vaccination.
- The neuraminidase inhibitors, oseltamivir and zanamivir, are the only antiviral medications recommended for chemoprophylaxis or treatment of influenza in children.

INTRODUCTION

Influenza causes significant morbidity and mortality every season. The 50 to 60 million cases each year result in approximately 25 million physician visits, 117,000 to 816,000 hospitalizations, and between 3,300 and 48,000 deaths. Mortality secondary to the influenza virus has been reported in chronically ill and previously healthy children. Invasive secondary infections or coinfections with group A streptococcus, *Staphylococcus aureus* (including methicillin-resistant *S aureus*), *Streptococcus pneumoniae*, or other bacterial pathogens can result in severe disease and death.

Most cases of influenza are resolved without serious complications for healthy persons between the ages of 2 and 65. However, these individuals can increase a community's disease burden and put vulnerable populations in danger of complications

Disclosure Statement: The authors declare no conflicts of interest.
a Division of Infectious Diseases, Department of Pediatrics, Children's Mercy Kansas City, 2401 Gillham Road, Kansas City, MO 64108, USA; b University of Missouri-Kansas City School of Medicine, 2411 Holmes Road, Kansas City, MO 64108, USA; c Department of Pediatrics, Cohen Children's Medical Center of NY, Hofstra Northshore-LIJ School of Medicine, 410 Lakeville Road, Suite 108, New Hyde Park, NY 11042, USA
* Corresponding author. Division of Infectious Diseases, Department of Pediatrics, Children's Mercy Kansas City, 2401 Gillham Road, Kansas City, MO 64108.
E-mail address: ralivingston@cmh.edu

Infect Dis Clin N Am 29 (2015) 597–615
http://dx.doi.org/10.1016/j.idc.2015.07.008
0891-5520/15/$ – see front matter © 2015 Elsevier Inc. All rights reserved.

from infection leading to hospitalization or even death. Vulnerable pediatric populations include children with high-risk conditions, such as hemoglobinopathies, chronic lung disease, asthma, cystic fibrosis, malignancy, diabetes mellitus, chronic renal disease, and congenital heart disease. Many complications, including death, may be prevented by annual influenza immunization.

INCIDENCE AND MORTALITY RATES

Influenza infects approximately 5% to 20% of children annually with school-aged children having the highest attack rates during pandemic and nonpandemic influenza seasons.[1,2] Children are the primary introducers of influenza into households with a secondary attack rate of 15% to 25% and are important vectors of influenza transmission in the community.[3] School holidays may impact transmission with secondary peaks in infection occurring once school resumes.

Pediatric mortality caused by influenza infection has been a nationally notifiable condition since 2004. On average, influenza causes 100 pediatric deaths per influenza season (Table 1). However, during the 2009 H1N1 influenza pandemic, which lasted from April 15, 2009 to October 2, 2010, a total of 348 pediatric deaths were reported to the Centers for Disease Control and Prevention (CDC).[4] In one study of 794 US children who died from influenza (median age, 7 years) between 2004 to 2005 through the 2011 to 2012 influenza seasons, 43% had no high-risk condition. Among the 57% that had one or more high-risk medical conditions, neurologic disorders were the most common condition reported (33%), followed by pulmonary disorders including asthma (26%), chromosome or genetic abnormalities (12%), and congenital or other type of cardiac disease (11%).[5] This study emphasizes that previously healthy children and those with underlying high-risk conditions are at risk for influenza death.

PATIENT HISTORY

Influenza is typically spread from person to person by large-particle respiratory tract droplets that are transmitted via coughing or sneezing. Contact with contaminated surfaces is another possible mode of transmission. Symptoms of influenza typically

Table 1
Pediatric deaths and hospitalizations by season and predominant strain

Influenza Season	Predominant Strain	Pediatric Deaths	Hospitalizations (0–4 y Old) Per 100,000	Hospitalizations (5–17 y Old) Per 100,000
2014–2015[a]	H3N2	145	58.3	16.9
2013–2014	pH1N1	111	47.3	9.4
2012–2013	H3N2	171	67	14.6
2011–2012[a]	H3N2	37	16	4
2010–2011	H3N2	123	49.5	9.1
2009–2010	pH1N1	288	77.4	27.2
2008–2009	H1N1	137	28	5
2007–2008	H3N2	88	40.3	5.5
2006–2007	H1N1	77	34.6	2.3
2005–2006	H3N2	46	28	4

[a] Vaccine strains did not change from previous influenza season.
From Centers for Disease Control and Prevention. FluView 2014–2015. Available at: http://www.cdc.gov/flu/weekly/fluviewinteractive.htm. Accessed August 14, 2015.

develop between 1 and 4 days after exposure (average, 2 days) and are listed in **Box 1**. Most symptoms peak by Day 2 of illness and continue to resolve over the next 1 to 2 weeks.

Other symptoms of influenza infection include congestion, sneezing, anorexia, malaise, and myositis. Conjunctivitis and gastrointestinal tract symptoms are more common in younger children than adults.[6] Young infants may present with symptoms similar to bacterial sepsis, and influenza infection has been associated with apnea in neonates.[7] Severe bilateral calf pain associated with difficulty walking can occur in the early convalescent phase of illness and is more commonly seen with influenza B infections.[8]

Peak viral shedding occurs on the day of symptom onset and declines steadily over the following week in adults.[9] Immunocompromised patients and children may shed virus for longer periods.[10,11] Individuals infected with influenza may be clinically asymptomatic but still shed virus and are capable of infecting others.

PHYSICAL EXAMINATION

Physical examination findings of influenza infection can overlap with many other causes of upper respiratory tract infections. The presence of wheezing, rhonchi, and/or rales suggests concomitant lower respiratory tract involvement. Multiple systems can be involved in more complicated disease presentations. **Box 2** lists physical examination findings by system that can be elicited from a patient suspected of having influenza.

During the 2014 to 2015 influenza season, multiple states notified the CDC of laboratory-confirmed influenza in persons presenting with parotitis. Of these reported cases most have occurred in children diagnosed with influenza A (H3) infection resulting in mild illness. Although parotitis associated with influenza A infection has been previously reported during the 1975 to 1976 and 1984 to 1985 influenza seasons, it remains an uncommon symptom associated with influenza infection.[12,13]

ADDITIONAL TESTING AND IMAGING

The early identification of influenza can reduce the amount of additional testing, decrease antibiotic use, and increase the use of appropriate antivirals. However, the

---

Box 1
Common signs and symptoms of influenza infection in children

- Fever (90%–97%)

- Dry nonproductive cough (77%–93%)

- Rhinitis (63%–78%)

- Pharyngitis (10%–36%)

- Headache (13%–26%)

- Conjunctivitis (9%)

- Nausea/vomiting/diarrhea (9%–15%)

- Myalgias (7%)

Frequency of symptoms noted in parentheses.

Data from Peltola V, Ziegler T, Ruuskanen O. Influenza A and B virus infections in children. Clin Infect Dis 2003;36:299–305; and Silvennoinen H, Peltola V, Lehtinen P, et al. Clinical presentation of influenza in unselected children treated as outpatients. Pediatr Infect Dis J 2009;28:372–5.

Box 2		
Physical exam findings of influenza infection		
General	**Cardiac**	**Gastrointestinal**
Fever	Tachycardia	Vomiting
Chills	Delayed capillary refill	Diarrhea
Sweating	Hemodynamic instability	
Rigors		
Head, Eyes, Ears, Nose,		
Throat (HEENT)	**Pulmonary**	**Neurologic**
Photophobia	Wheezing	Weakness
Eye pain with motion	Rhonchi	Fatigue
Conjuctivitis	Rales	Altered mental status
Otitis media	Tachypnea	Seizures
Congestion/rhinorrhea	Hypoxia	Ataxia
Hoarseness	Pleuritic chest pain	Coma
Pharyngeal inflammation		Myalgias
Cough		
Cervical lymphadenopathy		

case definition for influenza-like illness as set forth by the CDC (temperature $\geq$37.8°C, with cough and/or sore throat without a known cause other than influenza) has a moderate sensitivity of 64% to 65% and specificity of 67%.[14,15] Thus, many clinicians use additional testing methods to diagnose influenza.

Viral culture has historically been the gold standard for diagnosing influenza infection, but its turnaround time of 3 to 10 days to obtain results is typically too long to influence patient care. Shell vial cultures are processed more quickly, usually within 48 hours, and have similar accuracy to viral culture.[16] Recently, reverse-transcriptase polymerase chain reaction (RT-PCR) has replaced viral culture as the gold standard in influenza detection. RT-PCR is more sensitive than viral culture; has a typical processing time of 1 to 6 hours; and may have improved detection rates, up to 13% higher, as compared with culture.[17]

Rapid influenza diagnostic tests (RIDTs) are mostly immunoassays that detect influenza antigens. They detect and distinguish between influenza A and influenza B, detect but do not distinguish between influenza A and B, or detect only influenza A.[17] They are often used as point-of-care testing in medical offices, urgent care centers, and emergency departments because results are available in 30 minutes or less. However, reported sensitivities range from 10% to 80%, although specificity is often greater than 90%.[15] RIDTs should not be used outside of influenza season because positive tests are most likely to be false-positives during this period. A positive RIDT obtained outside of influenza season can be confirmed by viral culture or RT-PCR for those patients in whom there is a high index of suspicion.

Influenza infection can be tested for in respiratory specimens by direct/indirect immunofluorescence with results available in 1 to 4 hours. Sensitivities of influenza detection by this method range from 70% to 100% as compared with cell culture, which has a sensitivity of 100%.[17] Serologic testing is not recommended for diagnosis because antibodies are not detectable until 4 to 6 weeks after the onset of infection. PCR for influenza has higher sensitivity and specificity and use is targeted for those hospitalized and/or high-risk patients. A summary of influenza testing methods is described in **Table 2**.

Table 2
Comparison of types of influenza diagnostic tests

Influenza Diagnostic Test	Method	Availability	Typical Processing Time	Sensitivity	Distinguishing Subtype Strains of Influenza A	Cost
Rapid influenza diagnostic tests	Antigen detection	Wide	<30 min	10%–80%	No	$
Direct and indirect immunofluorescence assays	Antigen detection	Wide	1–4 h	70%–100%	No	$
Viral cell culture	Virus isolation	Limited	3–10 d	100%	Yes	$$
Rapid cell culture (shell vials and cell mixtures)	Virus isolation	Limited	1–3 d	100%	Yes	$$
Nucleic acid amplification tests (including rRT-PCR)	RNA detection	Limited	1–6 h	86%–100%	Yes	$$$
Rapid influenza molecular assays	RNA detection	Wide	<15 min	86%–100%	No	$$$

Adapted from the Centers for Disease Control and Prevention (CDC). Guidance for clinicians on the use of rapid influenza diagnostic tests. Available at: http://www.cdc.gov/flu/professionals/diagnosis/clinician_guidance_ridt.htm. Accessed June 30, 2015.

Data on hematologic manifestations of influenza infection in children are limited. A single center study involving 31 pediatric patients characterizing hematologic abnormalities in influenza A H1N1 infection divided study participants into three groups: no history of chronic disease (Group 1), underlying chronic disease other than a disease that may affect the bone marrow (Group 2), and underlying chronic disorder that may affect bone marrow including hematologic malignancies (Group 3).[18] Results are shown in **Table 3**.

Elevated creatinine kinase levels can be found in patients with associated influenza myositis.[8] Abnormal liver chemistries involving transaminases, γ-glutamyl transpeptidase, lactate dehydrogenase, bilirubin, prealbumin, total serum protein, and γ-globulin have been found in patients with influenza A H1N1.[19]

TREATMENT AND CHEMOPROPHYLAXIS

Two classes of antiviral drugs are available for the treatment/prophylaxis of influenza infection. The adamantanes, consisting of amantadine and ramantidine, are effective against influenza A but not influenza B. However, the adamantames are no longer recommended for use because of widespread levels of resistance in recently circulating influenza A (H3N2) strains. Influenza A 2009 H1N1 viral strains were also recently found to be resistant to the adamantanes.[20]

The neuraminidase inhibitors are effective against both influenza A and B. Three are approved by the US Food and Drug Administration for use: (1) oral oseltamivir (Tamiflu), (2) inhaled zanamivir (Relenza), and (3) intravenous peramivir (Rapivab). All three are available for the treatment of influenza A and B. However, only oseltamivir and zanamivir are approved for prophylaxis or treatment of influenza in children. Peramivir is administered as a single intravenous dose within 2 days of onset of influenza symptoms and is only approved for individuals 18 years of age and older.[21] Intravenous zanamivir is under investigation and only available to those enrolled in a clinical trial or by an emergency investigational new drug request. If an oseltamivir- or peramivir-resistant virus is a concern, use of intravenous zanamivir is recommended.

Table 4 provides recommended dosage and duration of antivirals for treatment and prophylaxis of influenza infection. Weight-based dosing of oseltamivir is not currently approved for the treatment of influenza in premature infants. The National Institute of Allergy and Infectious Diseases Collaborative Antiviral Study Group provides limited data on oseltamivir dosing recommendations for premature infants based on their postmenstrual age (gestational age + chronologic age; see footnote "c" in **Table 4**). For oseltamivir dosing recommendations in extremely premature infants (<28 weeks of age), consultation with a pediatric infectious disease expert is recommended.

Randomized controlled trials mostly in adults with mild illness in the outpatient setting have shown that either oseltamivir or zanamivir can decrease the duration of symptoms caused by influenza A and B by approximately 1 day when administered within 48 hours of onset of illness.[22] Two randomized controlled trials in pediatrics

Table 3
Hematologic abnormalities of patients with influenza A H1N1 according to underlying disorder

	Group 1 (N = 14)	Group 2 (N = 9)	Group 3 (N = 8)
Leukopenia, N (%)	2 (14.3)	1 (11.1)	5 (62.5)
Neutropenia, N (%)	2 (14.3)	2 (22.2)	6 (75)
Thrombocytopenia, N (%)	1 (7.1)	—	5 (62.5)

Table 4
Recommended dosage and schedule of influenza antiviral medications for treatment and chemoprophylaxis for the 2015–2016 influenza season: United States

Medication	Treatment (5 d)	Chemoprophylaxis (10 d)
Oseltamivir[a]		
Adults	75 mg twice daily	75 mg once daily
Children ≥12 mo		
Body wt		
≤15 kg (≤33 lb)	30 mg twice daily	30 mg once daily
>15–23 kg (33–51 lb)	45 mg twice daily	45 mg once daily
>23–40 kg (>51–88 lb)	60 mg twice daily	60 mg once daily
>40 kg (>88 lb)	75 mg twice daily	75 mg once daily
Infants 9–11 mo[b]	3.5 mg/kg per dose twice daily	3.5 mg/kg per dose once daily
Term infants 0–8 mo[b]	3 mg/kg per dose twice daily	3 mg/kg per dose once daily for infants 3–8 mo; not recommended for infants <3 mo old, unless situation judged critical, because of limited safety and efficacy data in this age group
Preterm infants	See details in footnote[c]	—
Zanamivir[d]		
Adults	10 mg (two 5-mg inhalations) twice daily	10 mg (two 5-mg inhalations) once daily
Children (≥7 y for treatment, ≥5 y for chemoprophylaxis)	10 mg (two 5-mg inhalations) twice daily	10 mg (two 5-mg inhalations) once daily

[a] Oseltamivir is administered orally without regard to meals, although administration with meals may improve gastrointestinal tolerability. Oseltamivir is available as Tamiflu in 30-, 45-, and 75-mg capsules and as a powder for oral suspension that is reconstituted to provide a final concentration of 6 mg/mL. For the 6-mg/mL suspension, a 30-mg dose is given with 5 mL of oral suspension, a 45-mg dose is given with 7.5 mL oral suspension, a 60-mg dose is given with 10 mL oral suspension, and a 75-mg dose is given with 12.5 mL oral suspension. If the commercially manufactured oral suspension is not available, a suspension can be compounded by retail pharmacies (final concentration also 6 mg/mL) based on instructions that are present in the package label. In patients with renal insufficiency, the dose should be adjusted based on creatinine clearance. For treatment of patients with creatinine clearance 10 to 30 mL/min: 75 mg, once daily, for 5 days. For chemoprophylaxis of patients with creatinine clearance 10 to 30 mL/min: 30 mg, once daily, for 10 days after exposure or 75 mg, once every other day, for 10 days after exposure (5 doses). See http://www.cdc.gov/flu/professionals/antivirals/antiviral-drug-resistance.htm.

[b] Approved by the Food and Drug Administration for children as young as 2 wk of age. Given preliminary pharmacokinetic data and limited safety data, oseltamivir can be used to treat influenza in term and preterm infants from birth because benefits of therapy are likely to outweigh possible risks of treatment.

[c] Oseltamivir dosing for preterm infants. The weight-based dosing recommendation for preterm infants is lower than for term infants. Preterm infants may have lower clearance of oseltamivir because of immature renal function, and doses recommended for full-term infants may lead to very high drug concentrations in this age group. Limited data from the National Institute of Allergy and Infectious Diseases Collaborative Antiviral Study Group provide the basis for dosing preterm infants using their postmenstrual age (gestational age + chronologic age): 1.0 mg/kg per dose, orally, twice daily, for those less than 38 wk postmenstrual age; 1.5 mg/kg per dose, orally, twice daily, for those 38 through 40 wk postmenstrual age; 3.0 mg/kg per dose, orally, twice daily, for those greater than 40 wk postmenstrual age. For extremely premature infants (<28 wk), consult a pediatric infectious diseases physician.

(continued on next page)

[d] Zanamivir is administered by inhalation using a proprietary "Diskhaler" device distributed together with the medication. Zanamivir is a dry powder, not an aerosol, and should not be administered using nebulizers, ventilators, or other devices typically used for administering medications in aerosolized solutions. Zanamivir is not recommended for people with chronic respiratory diseases, such as asthma or chronic obstructive pulmonary disease, which increase the risk of bronchospasm.

From Centers for Disease Control and Prevention. Antiviral agents for the treatment and chemoprophylaxis of influenza: recommendations of the Advisory Committee on Immunization Practices (ACIP). MMWR Recomm Rep 2011;60(RR-1):1–24; and Kimberlin DW, Acosta EP, Prichard MN, et al; National Institute of Allergy and Infectious Diseases Collaborative Antiviral Study Group. Oseltamivir pharmacokinetics, dosing, and resistance among children aged <2 years with influenza. J Infect Dis 2013;207(5):709–20.

of oseltamivir verses placebo showed a median reduction in symptoms of 1.5 and 3.5 days when oseltamivir was given within 48 hours and 24 hours of symptom onset, respectively, although no demonstration of efficacy against influenza B was seen with oseltamivir in the second study.[23,24] A trial of 346 children randomized to receive either zanamivir or placebo showed a reduction in symptoms of a median 1.25 days when subjects were given zanamivir within 36 hours of symptom onset.[25]

Certain individuals are at increased risk of developing complications from influenza infection and should receive treatment with an appropriate antiviral regardless of time since symptom onset (**Box 3**).

Antiviral treatment can be considered for previously healthy, symptomatic outpatients with confirmed or suspected influenza who are not considered high risk if treatment is started within 48 hours of illness onset.[26]

CLINICAL OUTCOMES AND COMPLICATIONS

Most children with influenza have mild infection and can be cared for in the outpatient setting with complete resolution of symptoms within 7 to 14 days. Children younger

---

Box 3
People at higher risk of influenza complications recommended for antiviral treatment of suspected or confirmed influenza

Children <2 y

Adults ≥65 y

People with chronic pulmonary (including asthma), cardiovascular (except hypertension alone), renal, hepatic, hematologic (including sickle cell disease), or metabolic disorders (including diabetes mellitus) or neurologic and neurodevelopment conditions (including disorders of the brain; spinal cord; peripheral nerve; and muscle, such as cerebral palsy, epilepsy [seizure disorders], stroke, intellectual disability [mental retardation], moderate to severe developmental delay, muscular dystrophy, or spinal cord injury)

People with immunosuppression, including that caused by medications or by HIV infection

Women who are pregnant or postpartum (within 2 wk after delivery)

People <19 y who are receiving long-term aspirin therapy

American Indian or Alaska Native people

People who are morbidly obese (ie, BMI ≥40)

Residents of nursing homes and other chronic care facilities

Data from Centers for Disease Control and Prevention. Antiviral agents for the treatment and chemoprophylaxis of influenza: recommendations of the Advisory Committee on Immunization (ACIP). MMWR Recomm Rep 2011;60(RR-1):1–24.

than 5 years of age, and especially those younger than 2 years of age, have the highest risk of complications from influenza and are hospitalized at an average rate of 60 per 100,000.[27] Complications range in severity from mild (ie, acute otitis media) to severe, including respiratory failure and death. The most common complications of influenza infection in children are described in **Table 5**.

Primary viral pneumonia is the least common of the pulmonary complications associated with influenza and has a mortality rate of 10% to 20% (**Fig. 1**).[28] Combined viral-bacterial pneumonia is three times as likely and has a similar mortality rate.[28] Secondary bacterial pneumonia has a mortality rate of approximately 7% and may be easier to diagnose because affected patients typically improve from their initial influenza illness and then deteriorate.[28] Secondary bacterial pneumonias are most frequently caused by infection with *S aureus*, including methicillin-resistant *S aureus*, *S pneumoniae* (the most common cause in children), *Haemophilus influenzae*, and *Streptococcus pyogenes* and are further complicated by the formation of empyemas and pneumatoceles (**Figs. 2** and **3**).

Influenza virus–associated encephalopathy is a disease that occurs mostly in young children between 6 and 18 months of age (**Fig. 4**).[29] Most cases have been reported in children from Japan and Taiwan but cases have also been reported in white children.[29] Clinical manifestations of influenza encephalopathy include seizures; altered mental status with coma and seizures; and mutism, a well described but less common neurologic manifestation. Most neurologic presentations occur on the day of or the day after influenza symptoms start. Reported case fatality rates are approximately 30%. Severe disability occurs in one-third of survivors and is associated with cerebral atrophy. A necrotizing encephalopathy occurs in approximately 20% of these children and is described as a symmetric necrosis of deep brain structures, resulting in death or disability in 70% of those affected.[29]

Table 5
Complications of influenza infection in children

Location	Complication	Frequency
Respiratory tract	Acute otitis media	9%
	Sinusitis	2%
	Bronchiolitis	7%
	Laryngotracheobronchitis (croup)	8%
	Pneumonia (viral or secondary bacterial)	12%
Cardiac	Myocarditis	0.4%
Central nervous system	Febrile seizures	9%
	Encephalitis/encephalopathy	2%
	Reye syndrome	a
	Guillain-Barré syndrome	b
	Transverse myelitis	b
	Aseptic meningitis	1%
Musculoskeletal	Myositis	23%

[a] Uncommon with one to two cases per year now that the link between salicylate use and Reye syndrome has been established.
[b] Unknown. Background rate of Guillain-Barré syndrome in children is 0.4 to 4 per 100,000.
Data from Peltola V, Ziegler T, Ruuskanen O. Influenza A and B virus infections in children. Clin Infect Dis 2003;36:299–305; and Moore DL, Vaudry W, Scheifele DW, et al. Surveillance for influenza admissions among children hospitalized in Canadian immunization monitoring program active centers, 2003–2004. Pediatrics 2006;118:e610–9.

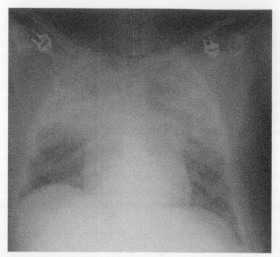

Fig. 1. Influenza pneumonia in a 12-year-old boy with respiratory failure. (*Courtesy of* Benjamin Estrada, MD.)

Reye syndrome occurs almost exclusively in children and is an acute illness characterized by encephalopathy and fatty degeneration of the liver. Symptoms include intense vomiting with neurologic manifestations that can progress to delirium, coma, and death.[30] Reye syndrome has been epidemiologically linked to the use of salicylates in the presence of infection with influenza and varicella. The number of reported cases peaked in 1980 at 555, but cases are now quite rare since warnings have been issued about the use of salicylates in children with viral infections and the risk of Reye syndrome.[31]

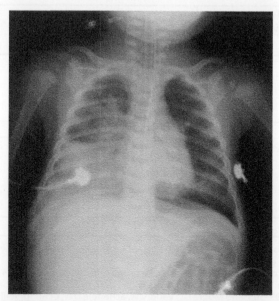

Fig. 2. Influenza A with *Staphylococcus aureus* pneumonia with empyema in a preschool-age child. (*Courtesy of* Benjamin Estrada, MD.)

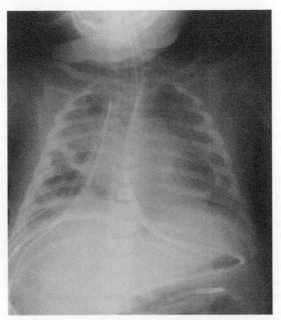

Fig. 3. Influenza A with *Staphylococcus aureus* superinfection in a 6 year old. Note the presence of bilateral pneumatoceles. (*Courtesy of* Benjamin Estrada, MD.)

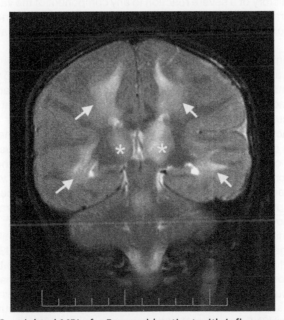

Fig. 4. Coronal T2-weighted MRI of a 5-year-old patient with influenza-associated encephalopathy demonstrating bilateral confluent signal hyperintensity in the white matter (*arrows*) and thalami (*asterisks*). (*Courtesy of* James Sejvar, MD.)

PREVENTION
Influenza Vaccine

Annual influenza vaccination of all children aged 6 months to 18 years is universally recommended by an increasing number of institutions, including the CDC, the American Academy of Pediatrics, and the American Academy of Family Physicians. Vaccine should be offered as soon as it becomes available for the season and continued as long as influenza viruses are circulating (**Table 6**). Children who require two doses in a given influenza season should receive their first dose as soon as possible and a second dose greater than or equal to 4 weeks later. Influenza vaccine is recommended for pregnant women at any point during pregnancy because they are at high risk for complications from influenza. This approach also provides protection for their infants during their first 6 months through transplacental transfer of antibodies. Children who turn 6 months of age during influenza season should be vaccinated. Both trivalent and quadrivalent influenza vaccines are available; neither formulation is preferred over the other.

Inactivated influenza vaccine (IIV) is approved for children 6 months of age and older. The most frequently reported side effect after IIV administration is pain at the injection site. Live attenuated influenza vaccine (LAIV) is approved for healthy children 2 years of age and older. Among children aged 2 to 17 years, the most frequently reported side effects after LAIV administration were runny nose/nasal congestion (32%) and fever greater than 100°F (7%).[32] Children diagnosed with asthma or children who are 5 years of age and younger who have had a medically attended wheezing episode in the previous 12 months or have a history of recurrent wheezing are not candidates for LAIV administration.[32] Children with egg allergy also are not candidates for LAIV administration. Recommendations for administering influenza vaccine in those who report egg allergy are detailed in **Fig. 5**. IIV and LAIV are contraindicated in children with a previous history of a severe reaction to any component of the vaccine. Additionally, LAIV is contraindicated in children and adolescents receiving concomitant aspirin therapy and should not be given to a child who is currently receiving an influenza antiviral agent.[32]

Two trivalent influenza vaccines manufactured using technologies that do not use eggs will also be available for people 18 years or older during the 2015 to 2016 season: cell culture–based IIV (ccIIV3, Flucelvax) and recombinant influenza vaccine (RIV3, FluBlok). The first vaccine, ccIIV3, is a trivalent cell culture–based IIV that is administered as an intramuscular injection and indicated for people 18 years or older. Although ccIIV3 is manufactured from virus propagated in cell culture rather than embryonated eggs, seed virus strains were created using virus strains that have been passaged in eggs. However, only trace amounts of ovalbumin are detectable and egg allergy is not listed as a contraindication in the package insert.[33] The second vaccine, RIV3, is a recombinant baculovirus-expressed hemagglutinin vaccine produced in cell culture. It is licensed for people 18 years or older and is administered via intramuscular injection. There are no egg proteins in this version of influenza vaccine.[34]

In one randomized, placebo-controlled trial of IIV and LAIV in children aged 1 to 15 years, vaccine was estimated to have 77% efficacy against H3N2 strains and 91% against H1N1 strains.[35] A randomized controlled trial of 1602 healthy children aged 15 to 71 months performed during two influenza seasons evaluated the efficacy of LAIV against culture-confirmed influenza. During the first season when vaccine and circulating strains were well matched, vaccine efficacy was 93%. During the second season when the H3N2 component of the vaccine was not well matched, vaccine efficacy was 86%.[36,37]

Table 6
Recommended seasonal influenza vaccines for different age groups: United States, 2015–2016 influenza season

Vaccine	Trade Name	Manufacturer	Presentation	Thimerosal Mercury Content (mm Hg/0.5-mL Dose)	Age Group
Inactivated					
IIV3	Fluzone	Sanofi Pasteur	0.5-mL prefilled syringe	0	≥36 mo
			5.0-mL multidose vial	25	≥6 mo
IIV3	Fluzone Intradermal	Sanofi Pasteur	0.1-mL prefilled microinjection	0	18–64 y
IIV3	Fluzone HD	Sanofi Pasteur	0.5-mL prefilled syringe	0	≥65 y
IIV3	Fluvirin	Novartis Vaccines and Diagnostics	0.5-mL prefilled syringe	≤1.0	≥4 y
			5.0-mL multidose vial	25	≥4 y
IIV3	Fluarix	GlaxoSmithKline	0.5-mL prefilled syringe	0	≥36 mo
IIV3	FluLaval	ID Biomedical Corporation of Quebec (distributed by GlaxoSmithKline)	0.5-mL prefilled syringe	0	≥36 mo
			5.0-mL multidose vial	<25	≥36 mo
IIV3	Afluria	bioCSL	0.5-mL prefilled syringe	0	≥9 y[a]
			5.0-mL multidose vial	24.5	≥9 y[a] via needle/syringe
					18–64 y via jet injector
ccIIV3	Flucelvax	Novartis Vaccines and Diagnostics	0.5-mL prefilled syringe	0	≥18 y

(continued on next page)

Table 6
(continued)

Vaccine	Trade Name	Manufacturer	Presentation	Thimerosal Mercury Content (mm Hg/0.5-mL Dose)	Age Group
IIV4	Fluzone Quadrivalent	Sanofi Pasteur	0.25-mL prefilled syringe	0	6–35 mo
			0.5-mL prefilled syringe	0	≥36 mo
			0.5-mL vial	0	≥36 mo
			5.0-mL multidose vial	25	≥6 mo
IIV4	Fluzone Intradermal Quadrivalent	Sanofi Pasteur	0.1-mL prefilled microinjection	0	18–64 y
IIV4	Fluarix Quadrivalent	GlaxoSmithKline	0.5-mL prefilled syringe	0	≥36 mo
IIV4	FluLaval Quadrivalent	ID Biomedical Corporation of Quebec (distributed by GlaxoSmithKline)	0.5-mL prefilled syringe	0	≥36 mo
			5.0-mL multidose vial	<25	≥36 mo
Recombinant					
RIV3	FluBlok	Protein Sciences	0.5-mL vial	0	≥18 y
Live attenuated					
LAIV4	FluMist Quadrivalent	MedImmune	0.2-mL sprayer	0	2–49 y

Abbreviations: ccIIV, cell culture–based inactivated influenza vaccine; IIV, inactivated influenza vaccine; LAIV, live attenuated influenza vaccine; RIV, recombinant influenza vaccine.

[a] Age indication per package insert is ≥5 years; however, the Advisory Committee on Immunization Practices recommends Afluria not be used in children 6 months through 8 years of age because of increased reports of febrile reactions noted in this age group. If no other age-appropriate, licensed inactivated seasonal influenza vaccine is available for a child 5 through 8 years of age who has a medical condition that increases the child's risk of influenza complications, Afluria can be used; however, pediatricians should discuss with the parents or caregivers the benefits and risks of influenza vaccination with Afluria before administering this vaccine.

Data from American Academy of Pediatrics; Committee on Infectious Diseases. Recommendations for prevention and control of influenza in children, 2014–2015. Pediatrics 2014;134(5):e1503–19; and Centers for Disease Control and Prevention. Prevention and control of seasonal influenza with vaccines: recommendations of the Advisory Committee on Immunization Practices (ACIP)—United States, 2015–2016 influenza season. MMWR Recomm Rep 2015;64(30);818–25.

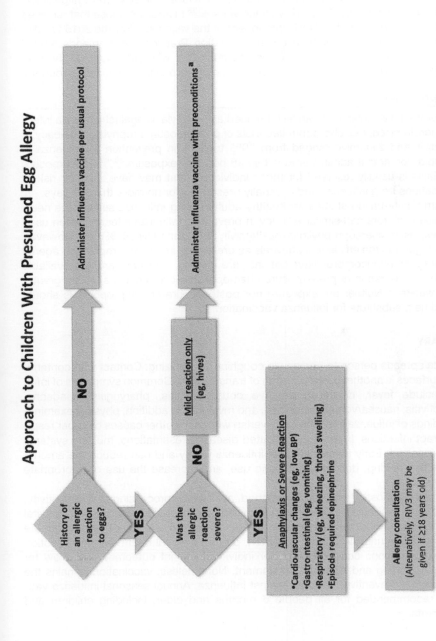

Approach to Children With Presumed Egg Allergy

History of an allergic reaction to eggs?

NO → Administer influenza vaccine per usual protocol

YES ↓

Was the allergic reaction severe?

NO (Mild reaction only [eg, hives]) → Administer influenza vaccine with preconditions [a]

YES ↓

Anaphylaxis or Severe Reaction
- Cardiovascular changes (eg, low BP)
- Gastrointestinal (eg, vomiting)
- Respiratory (eg, wheezing, throat swelling)
- Episodes required epinephrine

→ Allergy consultation (Alternatively, RIV3 may be given if ≥18 years old)

Fig. 5. Recommendations for influenza vaccination in those with presumed egg allergy. BP, blood pressure; RIV3, recombinant influenza vaccine, trivalent. [a] Necessary steps for administering influenza vaccine to any child with presumed egg allergy: in-office observation for 30 minutes; appropriate resuscitative equipment available. (*Data from* Erlewyn-Lajeunesse M, Brathwaite N, Lucas JS, et al. Recommendations for the administration of influenza vaccine in children allergic to egg. BMJ 2009;339:b3680.)

Influenza vaccine efficacy for the last three influenza seasons (2011–2012, 2012–2013, 2013–2014) has ranged from 52% to 61% for all age groups. However, vaccine effectiveness for the 2014 to 2015 season was estimated at only 19% for all age groups because 81% of circulating influenza A (H3N2) viruses was antigenically distinct from the influenza A (H3N2) vaccine viruses.[38] In addition, those that received LAIV did not respond to the H1N1 component of the vaccine.[38] For the 2015 to 2016 season, the Advisory Committee on Immunization Practices recommends annual influenza vaccination for everyone 6 months and older with either LAIV or IIV, with no preference expressed for either vaccine when either one is otherwise appropriate.

Chemoprophylaxis

The neuraminidase inhibitors can also be used as prophylaxis against influenza infection. In randomized, placebo-controlled trials of postexposure prophylaxis, efficacy of oseltamivir and zanamivir ranged from 79% to 84% in prevention of influenza in household contacts if administered within 48 hours of exposure.[39–41] Postexposure prophylaxis is usually reserved for those individuals that may have a higher risk of complications from influenza and is usually prescribed for no more than 10 days.

In community-based studies for healthy adults during influenza season the neuraminidase inhibitors had similar efficacy in preventing influenza infection when used as pre-exposure chemoprophylaxis (oseltamivir, 82%; zanamivir, 84%).[42,43] However, studies regarding the efficacy of antivirals as pre-exposure chemoprophylaxic agents in severely immunocompromised patients are lacking, and data are not available regarding the duration of pre-exposure chemoprophylactic regimens lasting greater than 6 weeks.[44] Neither pre-exposure nor postexposure chemoprophylaxis should be used as a substitute for influenza vaccination.

SUMMARY

Influenza spreads person to person via coughing or sneezing. Contact with contaminated surfaces is another possible mode of transmission. Common symptoms of influenza include fever, dry nonproductive cough, rhinitis, pharyngitis, headache, conjunctivitis, nausea/vomiting/diarrhea, and myalgias. In addition, physical examination findings of influenza infection can overlap with many other causes of upper respiratory tract infections. In more complicated disease presentations, multiple systems can be involved. Early identification of influenza is key and can reduce the amount of additional testing, decrease antibiotic use, and increase the use of appropriate antivirals.

Influenza diagnostic tests vary by method, availability, processing time, sensitivity, and cost, which should be considered in making the best clinical judgment. Antiviral medications are important in the control of influenza, but should not be a substitute for influenza immunization. Early detection, prompt antiviral treatment, and infection control interventions can lead to better individual patient outcomes and allow for effective cohorting and disease containment. Nonetheless, vaccination remains the best available preventive measure against influenza. Annual seasonal influenza vaccine is recommended for all people 6 months and older, including children and adolescents.

REFERENCES

1. Neuzil KM, Zhu Y, Griffin MR, et al. Burden of interpandemic influenza in children younger than 5 years: a 25-year prospective study. J Infect Dis 2002;185:147–52.

2. Glezen WP. Emerging infections: pandemic influenza. Epidemiol Rev 1996;18: 64–76.

3. Longini IM, Koopman JS, Monto AS, et al. Estimating household and community transmission parameters for influenza. Am J Epidemiol 1982;115:736–51.

4. 2013–2014 influenza season. Centers for Disease Control and Prevention. 2014. Available at: http://www.cdc.gov/flu/pastseasons/1314season.htm. Accessed April 21, 2015.

5. Wong KK, Jain S, Blanton L, et al. Influenza-associated pediatric deaths in the United States, 2004–2012. Pediatrics 2013;132:796–804.

6. Peltola V, Ziegler T, Ruuskanen O. Influenza A and B virus infections in children. Clin Infect Dis 2003;36:299–305.

7. Meibalane R, Sedmak GV, Sasidharan P, et al. Outbreak of influenza in a neonatal intensive care unit. J Pediatr 1977;91:974–6.

8. Hu JJ, Kao CL, Lee PI, et al. Clinical features of influenza A and B in children and association with myositis. J Microbiol Immunol Infect 2004;37:95–8.

9. Lau LL, Cowling BJ, Fang VJ, et al. Viral shedding and clinical illness in naturally acquired influenza virus infections. J Infect Dis 2010;201:1509–16.

10. Klimov AI, Rocha E, Hayden FG, et al. Prolonged shedding of amantadine-resistant influenza A viruses by immunodeficient patients: detection by polymerase chain reaction-restriction analysis. J Infect Dis 1995;172:1352–5.

11. Frank AL, Taber LH, Wells CR, et al. Patterns of shedding of myxoviruses and paramyxoviruses in children. J Infect Dis 1981;144:433–41.

12. Brill SJ, Gilfillan RF. Acute parotitis associated with influenza type A: a report of twelve cases. N Engl J Med 1977;296:1391–2.

13. Krilov LR, Swenson P. Acute parotitis associated with influenza A infection. J Infect Dis 1985;152:853.

14. Overview of influenza surveillance in the United States. Centers for Disease Control and Prevention. 2015. Available at: http://www.cdc.gov/flu/weekly/overview.htm. Accessed April 25, 2015.

15. Chartrand C, Leeflang MM, Minion J, et al. Accuracy of rapid influenza diagnostic tests: a meta-analysis. Ann Intern Med 2012;156:500–11.

16. Dunn JJ, Woolstenhulme RD, Langer J, et al. Sensitivity of respiratory virus culture when screening with R-mix fresh cells. J Clin Microbiol 2004;42:79–82.

17. WHO Recommendations on the use of rapid testing for influenza diagnosis. World Health Organization. 2005. Available at: http://www.who.int/influenza/resources/documents/RapidTestInfluenza_WebVersion.pdf?ua=1. Accessed May 10, 2015.

18. Ünal S, Gökce M, Aytac-Elmas S, et al. Hematological consequences of pandemic influenza H1N1 infection: a single center experience. Turk J Pediatr 2010;52:570–5.

19. Yingying C. Abnormal liver chemistry in patients with influenza A H1N1. Liver Int 2011;31:902.

20. Antiviral drugs for seasonal influenza: additional links and resources. Centers for Disease Control and Prevention. 2015. Available at: http://www.cdc.gov/flu/professionals/antivirals/links.htm. Accessed May 27, 2015.

21. Highlights of prescribing information: Rapivab (peramivir injection). Food and Drug Administration. 2014. Available at: http://www.accessdata.fda.gov/drugsatfda_docs/label/2014/206426lbl.pdf. Accessed May 27, 2015.

22. Fiore AE, Fry A, Shay D, et al, Centers for Disease Control and Prevention. Antiviral agents for the treatment and chemoprophylaxis of influenza—recommendations of the Advisory Committee on Immunization Practices (ACIP). MMWR Surveill Summ 2011;60:1–24.

23. Whitley RJ, Hayden FG, Reisinger KS, et al. Oral oseltamivir treatment of influenza in children. Pediatr Infect Dis J 2001;20:127–33.

24. Heinonen S, Silvennoinen H, Lehtinen P, et al. Early oseltamivir treatment of influenza in children 1–3 years of age: a randomized controlled trial. Clin Infect Dis 2010;51:887–94.

25. Hedrick JA, Barzilai A, Behre U, et al. Zanamivir for treatment of symptomatic influenza A and B infection in children five to twelve years of age: a randomized controlled trial. Pediatr Infect Dis J 2000;19(5):410–7.

26. Influenza antiviral medications: summary for clinicians. Centers for Disease Control and Prevention Web Site. 2015. Available at: http://www.cdc.gov/flu/professionals/antivirals/summary-clinicians.htm. Accessed July 1, 2015.

27. Iwane MK, Edwards KM, Szilagyi PG, et al. Population-based surveillance for hospitalizations associated with respiratory syncytial virus, influenza virus, and parainfluenza viruses among young children. Pediatrics 2004;113:1758–64.

28. Metersky ML, Masterton RG, Lode H, et al. Epidemiology, microbiology, and treatment considerations for bacterial pneumonia complicating influenza [review]. Int J Infect Dis 2012;16:e321–31.

29. Surtees R, DeSousa C. Influenza virus associated encephalopathy. Arch Dis Child 2006;91:455–6.

30. Centers for Disease Control and Prevention. Reye syndrome surveillance—United States, 1989. MMWR Morb Mortal Wkly Rep 1991;40:88–90.

31. Belay ED, Bresee JS, Holman RC, et al. Reye's syndrome in the United States from 1981 through 1997. N Engl J Med 1999;340:1377–82.

32. Highlights of prescribing information: Flumist quadrivalent. Medimmune. Available at: http://www.medimmune.com/docs/default-source/default-document-library/product-and-patient-information-for-flumist-quadrivalent.pdf. Accessed July 5, 2015.

33. FLUCELVAX - Novartis Vaccines and Diagnostics, Inc 1.14.1.3 US Package Insert April 2015. Food and Drug Administration. Available at: http://www.fda.gov/downloads/BiologicsBloodVaccines/Vaccines/ApprovedProducts/UCM329134.pdf. Accessed July 5, 2015.

34. Protein Sciences Corporation Influenza Vaccine Package Insert BLA STN 125285. Available at: http://www.fda.gov/downloads/BiologicsBloodVaccines/Vaccines/ApprovedProducts/UCM336020.pdf. Accessed July 5, 2015.

35. Neuzil KM, Dupont WD, Wright PF, et al. Efficacy of inactivated and cold-adapted vaccines. against influenza A infection, 1985 to 1990: the pediatric experience. Pediatr Infect Dis J 2001;20:733–40.

36. Belshe RB, Mendelman PM, Treanor J, et al. The efficacy of live attenuated, cold-adapted, trivalent, intranasal influenza virus vaccine in children. N Engl J Med 1998;338:1405–12.

37. Belshe RB, Edwards KM, Vesikari T, et al, CAIV-T Comparative Efficacy Study Group. Live attenuated versus inactivated influenza vaccine in infants and young children. N Engl J Med 2007;356:685–96.

38. Centers for Disease Control and Prevention. Update: influenza activity—United States, September 28, 2014-February 21, 2015. MMWR Morb Mortal Wkly Rep 2015;64:206–12.

39. Hayden FG, Gubareva LV, Monto AS, et al, Zanamivir Family Study Group. Inhaled zanamivir for the prevention of influenza in families. N Engl J Med 2000;343:1282–9.

40. Welliver R, Monto AS, Carewicz O, et al, Oseltamivir Post Exposure Prophylaxis Investigator Group. Effectiveness of oseltamivir in preventing influenza in household contacts: a randomized controlled trial. JAMA 2001;285:748–54.

41. Monto AS, Pichichero ME, Blanckenberg SJ, et al. Zanamivir prophylaxis: an effective strategy for the prevention of influenza types A and B within households. J Infect Dis 2002;186(11):1582–8.
42. Hayden FG, Atmar RL, Schilling M, et al. Use of the selective oral neuraminidase inhibitor oseltamivir to prevent influenza. N Engl J Med 1999;341:1336–43.
43. Monto AS, Robinson DP, Herlocher ML, et al. Zanamivir in the prevention of influenza among healthy adults: a randomized controlled trial. JAMA 1999;282:31–5.
44. Khazeni N, Bravata DM, Holty JE, et al. Systematic review: safety and efficacy of extended-duration antiviral chemoprophylaxis against pandemic and seasonal influenza. Ann Intern Med 2009;151:464–73.

Rotavirus Infection
A Disease of the Past?

Penelope H. Dennehy, MD

KEYWORDS

- Rotavirus • Rotavirus vaccine • Rotavirus gastroenteritis • Rotavirus surveillance
- Rotavirus immunity

KEY POINTS

- Rotavirus vaccination had been implemented in national vaccination programs in 77 countries worldwide.
- Rotavirus vaccines have reduced the burden of rotavirus disease in the United States and other high- and middle-income countries.
- The real-world effectiveness data for both vaccines are consistent with efficacy data obtained from clinical trials.
- Herd immunity has also been seen after vaccine introduction.
- Vaccine introduction has led to no significant strain shifts or escape mutants as yet.

ROTAVIRUS DISEASE BURDEN

Rotavirus infection is the leading cause of severe acute diarrhea among children less than 5 years of age worldwide, causing an estimated

- 453,000 deaths each year, with greater than 85% of these deaths occurring in low-income countries of Africa and Asia [1]
- 5% of all deaths worldwide[1]
- 114 million episodes of gastroenteritis requiring only home care, 24 million clinic visits, and 2.4 million hospitalizations[2]
- 36% of all diarrhea hospitalizations[3]

The public health burden of rotavirus was confirmed by the Global Enteric Multicenter Study (GEMS), the first comprehensive global study of childhood diarrheal disease, which was conducted in 7 study sites in sub-Saharan Africa and South Asia.

Dr P.H. Dennehy has received research grants from Merck and GlaxoSmithKline Biologicals.
Division of Pediatric Infectious Diseases, Department of Pediatrics, Hasbro Children's Hospital, 593 Eddy Street, Providence, RI 02903, USA
E-mail address: pdennehy@lifespan.org

Infect Dis Clin N Am 29 (2015) 617–635
http://dx.doi.org/10.1016/j.idc.2015.07.002
0891-5520/15/$ – see front matter © 2015 Elsevier Inc. All rights reserved.

id.theclinics.com

GEMS found that rotavirus is the overall leading cause of moderate to severe diarrhea among infants and toddlers less than 2 years of age and a major cause among children less than 5 years of age in these settings.[4]

In the United States before the introduction of rotavirus vaccine in 2006, 95% of children experienced at least one rotavirus infection by age 5 years.[5] A significant illness burden was attributable to rotavirus gastroenteritis, including an estimated

- 20 to 60 deaths, 55,000 to 70,000 hospitalizations, more than 200,000 emergency department visits, and more than 400,000 outpatient visits annually[6]
- 5% to 10% of all gastroenteritis episodes among children less than 5 years of age[7]
- 30% to 50% of all hospitalizations for gastroenteritis among children aged less than 5 years, and more than 70% of hospitalizations for gastroenteritis during the seasonal peaks of rotavirus disease[7]
- Annual direct and indirect costs of approximately $1 billion, primarily because of the cost of time lost from work to care for an ill child[8,9]

CLINICAL ASPECTS OF ROTAVIRUS DISEASE

The clinical manifestations of infection vary and depend on whether risk factors for severe disease are present (**Box 1**). Rotavirus predominantly infects children, but infection also occurs in adults.

Box 1
Risk factors for severe rotavirus disease

Primary infection

- Initial infection after age 3 months is most likely to cause severe diarrhea and dehydration.

Age

- In industrialized countries, severe, dehydrating rotavirus gastroenteritis primarily occurs among infants and children aged 3 to 35 months, although 25% of cases of severe disease occur after 2 years of age.

- In resource-poor countries, the vast proportion of severe rotavirus disease (60%–80%) occurs by 12 to 15 months of age.

Preterm birth

- Most mothers have rotavirus antibody from previous infection that is passed transplacentally, protecting the neonate. As a result, most infected neonates will have asymptomatic or mild disease.

- An exception is the preterm infant, who is at greater risk of severe illness than the term infant because of the lack of transplacental maternal antibodies.

Immunodeficiencies

- Severe and prolonged rotavirus gastroenteritis has been reported in children with T-cell immunodeficiencies or severe combined immunodeficiency, and after bone marrow transplantation.

- Infection of children after solid organ transplantation is usually self-limited but more severe than in healthy children.

- Rotavirus does not seem to be a common cause of severe or persistent diarrhea in individuals with human immunodeficiency virus infection.

Studies of children with rotavirus infection have shown a spectrum of disease, ranging from asymptomatic shedding to severe dehydration, seizures, and even death. Following a short incubation period (1–3 days), rotavirus gastroenteritis usually begins with abrupt onset of fever and vomiting followed 24 to 48 hours later by watery diarrhea (**Box 2**).[10] Symptoms generally persist for 3 to 8 days, although protracted episodes have been noted on occasion.

Dehydration and electrolyte disturbances are the major sequelae of rotavirus infection and occur most often in the youngest children. Studies of hospitalized children have indicated that cases of gastroenteritis associated with rotavirus have tended to be more severe than cases in which rotavirus was not detected, with more severe dehydration and higher incidences of vomiting and fever.[7]

No antiviral is currently available to treat rotavirus infection. The current mainstay of treatment of acute rotavirus gastroenteritis consists of oral rehydration and early introduction of feedings. Adequate fluid and electrolyte replacement and maintenance are the key to managing rotavirus gastroenteritis.

EPIDEMIOLOGY OF ROTAVIRUS DISEASE

Rotavirus is ubiquitous worldwide. The epidemiology of rotavirus is detailed in **Box 3**.

PROSPECTS OF ERADICATION OF ROTAVIRUS DISEASE

The fact that infection with rotavirus is universal so early in childhood indicates the virus is not primarily transmitted via fecally contaminated water or food, distinguishing it from other major causes of viral, bacterial, or parasitic causes of gastroenteritis. Given the major contribution of rotavirus to the global disease burden caused by diarrheal diseases and the fact that improvements in economic development are unlikely to greatly impact disease incidence, vaccination is the primary strategy of control.

Prevention of Rotavirus Infection Through Vaccination

A realistic goal for a rotavirus vaccine is to duplicate the degree of protection against disease that follows natural infection (**Box 4**). Therefore, vaccine program objectives

---

Box 2
Typical symptoms of rotavirus infection in children

Fever

- Occurs in up to half of all infected children

- Usually low grade

- Up to a third of infected children may have a temperature greater than 102°F (39°C), which may trigger seizures in children with a propensity for febrile seizures

Vomiting

- Nonbilious

- Occurs in 80% to 90% of infected children

- Usually brief, lasting 24 hours or less in most children

Diarrhea

- Watery, nonbloody

- On average up to 10 to 20 bowel movements per day

- Persists for 3 to 8 days

> **Box 3**
> **Epidemiology of rotavirus disease**
>
> *Reservoir*
>
> - The gastrointestinal tract and stool of infected humans
> - Transmission of animal rotaviruses to humans is thought to be rare and probably does not lead to clinical illness
> - A true carrier state has not been described
>
> *Communicability*
>
> - This virus is highly communicable with a small infectious dose of less than 100 viral particles.
> - Infected persons shed large quantities of virus in their stool beginning 2 days before the onset of diarrhea and for up to 10 days after onset of symptoms.
> - Virus spreads easily from person to person through contaminated hands and objects, such as toys and surfaces. Rotavirus can live on contaminated hands for hours and surfaces for days.
> - Rotavirus spread within families, institutions, hospitals, and child care settings is common.
>
> *Mode of transmission*
>
> - Primarily by the fecal-oral route through person-to-person contact or by fomites
> - Possibly by aerosolized respiratory droplets, as suggested by the seasonality seen in temperate climates (similar to influenza, respiratory syncytial virus, and measles)
> - Rare common-source outbreaks from contaminated water or food
>
> *Seasonality*
>
> - As with other respiratory and enteric viruses, rotavirus disease is associated with distinct seasonality.
> - In temperate climates, disease is most prevalent during the cooler months.
>   - Before licensure of rotavirus vaccines in North America, the annual epidemic usually started during the autumn in Mexico and the southwest United States and moved eastward, reaching the northeast United States and Canada by spring.
>   - A similar pattern exists in Europe, with the seasonal peak beginning in Spain in January, spreading to northern countries by March.
> - The seasonal pattern of disease is less pronounced in tropical climates, with rotavirus infection being more common during the cooler, drier months.
> - The reason for this seasonality remains unknown.

include the prevention of moderate to severe disease but not necessarily of mild disease associated with rotavirus. An effective rotavirus vaccine will clearly decrease the number of children admitted to the hospital with dehydration or seen in emergency departments, but should also decrease the burden on the practicing primary care practitioner by reducing the number of office visits or telephone calls due to rotavirus gastroenteritis. Eradication of rotavirus disease is unlikely because mild infections will continue to occur, providing a continued although reduced reservoir of virus in the community.

Rotavirus Strain Diversity

Implementation of an effective rotavirus vaccine program will need to take into account the geographic variation of prevalent strains. Rotavirus strains are defined by 2 surface proteins, VP7 (a glycoprotein, G protein) and VP4 (a protease-cleaved

---

Box 4
Immunity to rotavirus infection and disease

Unlike other viral infections, such as measles, rotavirus infection normally provides short-term protection and immunity against severe subsequent illness but not lifelong immunity.[76]

After a single natural infection[77]:

- 38% of children are protected against any subsequent rotavirus infection

- 77% are protected against rotavirus diarrhea

- 87% are protected against severe diarrhea

Subsequent infections

- Occur at any age

- Confer progressively greater protection

- Generally less severe than the first

Immune correlates of protection[76]

- Poorly understood despite 4 decades of research

- Serum and mucosal antibodies against viral surface proteins VP7 and VP4 are probably important for protection from disease

- Cell-mediated immunity probably plays a role in recovery from infection and in protection.

---

protein, P protein), found in the outer capsid of the virus. These 2 proteins define the serotype of the virus and are targets for neutralizing antibodies that may provide both homotypic and heterotypic protection. At least 12 G types and 15 P types have been identified in humans.

Rotavirus is capable of substantial genetic diversity because the virus has a segmented genome that can undergo gene reassortment. The ability of the virus to mutate and reassort allows for the potential of new and emerging serotypes of rotaviruses. Reassortment alone could theoretically lead to almost 200 different G and P combinations. However, although greater than 60 G-P combinations have been found in humans, 5 strains are most commonly associated with human disease worldwide (G1P[8], G2P[4], G3P[8], G4P[8], and G9P[8]). These strains are responsible for 80% to 90% of the childhood rotavirus disease burden globally.[11] The G2P[4] rotavirus strain belongs to a different G serotype, P subtype, and genogroup than the other globally common strains. Circulating strains vary both regionally and temporally with substantial year-to-year, seasonal, and geographic variability. In addition, multiple strains can circulate within the same region at the same time. The continued identification of the most common G and P serotypes for inclusion in vaccines is an important priority. After introduction of a vaccine, monitoring of circulating strains is necessary, because vaccine pressure may lead to the selection of novel rotavirus strains

Rotavirus Vaccine Development Strategies

Rotavirus vaccine development began shortly after human rotavirus was identified in 1973. To date, all rotavirus vaccines tested in children have been either live oral viral vaccines developed by a Jennerian or modified Jennerian approach or using attenuated human rotaviruses (**Table 1**).

The earliest vaccine candidates were developed using what has been called the Jennerian approach, applying Edward Jenner's concept of using animal strains, which were observed to be naturally attenuated, to induce protection against human strains.

Table 1
Rotavirus vaccine development strategies

Strategy	Parent Rotavirus	Vaccine Name (Serotypes)	Efficacy	Current Use	Location
Monovalent animal vaccine	Bovine	RIT 4237 (P6[1]G6)	Low	No	—
	Bovine	WC3 (P7[5]G6)	Low	No	—
	Simian (rhesus)	MMU1006 (P5B[3] G3)	Low	No	—
	Lamb	LLR (P[12]G10)	Moderate	Yes	China
Multivalent human–animal reassortant vaccines	Simian (rhesus)	RRV-TV (P7[5]G1-4) RotaShield	High	No (withdrawn due to intussusception risk)	United States
	Bovine	RV5 (P1A[8]G1-4) RotaTeq	High	Yes	Worldwide
Naturally occurring human–bovine reassortant vaccine	Human	116E (P[10]G9) ROTAVAC	High	Yes	India
Live-attenuated human vaccine	Human	RV1 (P1A[8]G1) Rotarix	High	Yes	Worldwide

Three animal rotavirus strains, 2 bovine, and a simian (rhesus) strain were studied as possible human vaccines. These vaccines demonstrated variable efficacy in field trials and gave particularly disappointing results in resource-poor countries and were not developed further. In 2000, China introduced the Lanzhou lamb rotavirus (LLR) vaccine, a monovalent live-attenuated oral vaccine that was derived from a lamb strain of rotavirus, for childhood immunization.[12] This vaccine is currently in use in China.

In view of the inconsistency of protection from monovalent animal rotavirus–based vaccines, vaccine development efforts shifted to take advantage of the ability of rotaviruses to reassort to produce novel reassortant vaccines that contained immunologically important proteins from human rotaviruses (VP7) and other genes from the animal strain to maintain the attenuated aspect, the so-called modified Jennerian approach. Furthermore, with a better understanding of the existence and distribution of rotavirus G serotypes, the second-generation vaccines were formulated to attempt to broaden immunity across serotypes by including several human G serotypes.

The first multivalent live oral reassortant vaccine developed was rhesus rotavirus-tetravalent vaccine (RRV-TV, Rotashield). RRV-TV is a quadrivalent vaccine based on the attenuated phenotype of the rhesus rotavirus and contains the 4 most common circulating human G serotypes: G1, G2, G3, and G4. Efficacy trials of RRV-TV demonstrated a high level of protection (80%–100%) in preventing severe diarrheal disease.[13] The RRV-TV vaccine was licensed in August 1998 for routine use in children in the United States. After inclusion of this vaccine in the immunization schedule in the United States,[14] and immunization of more than 600,000 infants in the first 9 months of the program, several cases of vaccine-associated intussusception were reported.[15] The period of greatest risk of intussusception was shown to be 3 to 10 days after the first of 3 oral doses.[16] Although the true overall incidence of this adverse event proved difficult to assess, a group of international experts suggested a consensus rate of 1 per 10,000 vaccinated infants.[17] The pathogenic mechanisms involved in intussusception following vaccination are currently unknown. As a consequence of this rare but potentially dangerous adverse effect, RRV-TV was withdrawn from the market in the United States.[18]

Following the withdrawal of RRV-TV, subsequent development focused on human–bovine reassortant strains or attenuated human strains. The human–bovine reassortant rotavirus strains include either human VP7 or VP4 genes. Initially, VP7 was thought to be the most important antigen in inducing protection; therefore, human–animal reassortant strains, such as those in RRV-TV, included only human VP7 genes to provide protective immune responses. More recently, VP4 has also been considered important in protection. Human–animal reassortant rotavirus strains now include either human VP7 or VP4 genes to provide protective immune responses. Using the previously tested bovine rotavirus strain (WC3) as a backbone, researchers created a pentavalent vaccine, RV5 (RotaTeq), containing 5 human–bovine reassortant rotavirus strains: 4 expressing human G1, G2, G3, G4, and bovine (WC3) P7[5] and one reassortant expressing P1A[8] (human) and G6 (bovine). RV5 was licensed following successful trials showing safety, immunogenicity, and efficacy.[19,20]

Various observational studies have suggested that neonatal rotavirus infection confers protection against diarrhea due to subsequent rotavirus infection. A strain obtained from asymptomatically infected newborns in India (116E) has been assessed as vaccine candidate. The116E vaccine is a naturally occurring human–bovine reassortant P[11]G9 strain with a single bovine gene segment encoding VP4. This vaccine was safe and efficacious in Indian infants[21,22] and was licensed as ROTAVAC. This vaccine has been available for use in children in India since January 2014.

The observation that the first natural rotavirus infection, either symptomatic or asymptomatic, provides protective immunity against subsequent severe disease, irrespective of serotype, was the underlying logic behind the approach of developing a live-attenuated human strain vaccine. RV1 (Rotarix) was developed using a wild-type human rotavirus P1A[8]G1 strain that represented the most common human rotavirus VP7 and VP4 antigens.[23] The vaccine was attenuated by multiple tissue culture passages. RV1 was licensed following successful trials showing safety, immunogenicity, and efficacy.[24,25]

Results of Clinical Trials of Rotavirus Vaccines

Efficacy of rotavirus vaccines in clinical trials has ranged from 72% to 100% in high- and middle-income countries with low mortalities[19,24,26,27] to 46% to 72% in low-income countries with high child mortalities.[28–30] Trials in the developing countries of Africa and Asia have shown lower efficacy of the vaccines but a larger absolute number of severe cases of rotavirus prevented through vaccination.[28–30] Given the high rates of rotavirus infection in resource-limited areas, use of these vaccines has the potential to dramatically decrease severe disease and mortality despite lower vaccine efficacy.

Efficacy of both RV1 and RV5 in preventing rotavirus diarrhea was assessed in a recent Cochrane Review.[31] Forty-three trials were included in the review: 31 assessing RV1 and 12 evaluating RV5. The review found that RV1 and RV5 vaccines are effective in preventing rotavirus diarrhea, with the data supporting the global vaccine recommendation by the World Health Organization (WHO; **Table 2**). Reported serious adverse events (including intussusception) after vaccination were measured in 95,178 children for RV1 and 77,480 for RV5, with no difference between the vaccines.

Table 2
Results of the 2012 *Cochrane Review* of rotavirus vaccine clinical trials

	Age at Vaccination			
	First Year of Life		Second Year of Life	
	Vaccine		Vaccine	
	RV1	RV5	RV1	RV5
Disease	% Prevented	% Prevented	% Prevented	% Prevented
All rotavirus diarrhea cases	70	73	70	49
Severe rotavirus diarrhea cases	80	77	84	56
Rotavirus diarrhea cases that require hospitalization	>80	>80	n/a	n/a
Severe cases of all-cause diarrhea	42	72	51	0

Abbreviation: n/a, not available.

AVAILABLE ROTAVIRUS VACCINES

Currently available rotavirus vaccines are shown in **Table 3**. Other new rotavirus vaccines are being developed by manufacturers in India, China, and Brazil and may be available soon.

Recommendations for Use of the Licensed Rotavirus Vaccines

RV1 and RV5 are recommended for routine immunization of all infants by the WHO.[32] In 2013, the WHO recommended inclusion of rotavirus vaccines in all national immunization programs, especially in countries with high rotavirus gastroenteritis-associated fatality rates, such as in south and south-eastern Asia and sub-Saharan Africa.[33] Both vaccines are also recommended for routine immunization of all infants in the United States by the Centers for Disease Control and Prevention (CDC) and the American Academy of Pediatrics.[7,34]

Currently, rotavirus vaccines are part of the national immunization program in 77 (40%) of 193 countries worldwide. Other countries, such as Canada and Thailand, have introduced rotavirus vaccines in pilot or regional introductions. Rotavirus vaccines are also available in more than 100 countries through the private market. With

Table 3
Available rotavirus vaccines

Global Market	National Markets
RV1 Rotarix (GlaxoSmithKline) FDA licensed in April 2008, The European Commission and the European Medicines Agency (EMA) licensed in February 2006, and WHO prequalified in January 2007	*116E* ROTAVAC (Bharat Biotech International Limited) licensed for use in India in 2014
RV5 RotaTeq (Merck & Co, Inc) FDA licensed in February 2006, EMA licensed in June 2006, and WHO prequalified in October 2008	*Rotavin-M1* (the Center for Research and Production of Vaccines) licensed for use in Vietnam in 2007
—	*LLR* Lanzhou Lamb Rotavirus Vaccine (Lanzhou Institute of Biological Products) licensed for use in China in 2000

donor support, the GAVI Alliance (formerly the Global Alliance for Vaccines and Immunisations) has introduced rotavirus vaccine in 35 low-income countries.

Each country has its own immunization schedule. The 2 rotavirus vaccines differ in the number of doses given. In general, in low-income countries, RV5 is given in 3 doses at 6 weeks, 10 weeks, and 14 weeks of age, and RV1 is given in 2 doses at 6 weeks and 10 weeks of age. In middle- and upper-income countries, RV5 is given in 3 doses at 2 months, 4 months, and 6 months of age, and RV1 is given in 2 doses at 2 months and 4 months of age. Differences in rotavirus immunization schedules are generally due to existing routine immunization program schedules and the logistics of delivering multiple vaccines at the same time.

In many low-income countries, because of challenges related to health service access, children may not receive their vaccines on schedule. WHO recommends in its 2013 rotavirus position paper that countries consider providing rotavirus vaccination to these children even if later than the immunization schedule specifies because the benefits of rotavirus vaccination, including preventing hospitalizations and deaths from diarrhea, far exceed any possible low-level risks associated with the vaccine (such as intussusception).[33]

Evaluation of the Safety Profile of Rotavirus Vaccine After Licensure

RV1 and RV5 were not associated with intussusception in large prelicensure trials.[19,24] In the United States, some, but not all, after-licensure studies suggest that RV5 and RV1 vaccines may possibly cause a small increase in the risk of intussusception. It is possible that an estimated 1 to 3 US infants of 100,000 immunized might develop intussusception within 7 days of getting their first dose of rotavirus vaccine.[35–38] That means 40 to 120 vaccinated US infants might develop intussusception each year. The benefits of rotavirus vaccines in preventing hospitalizations and deaths from rotavirus illness far outweigh the small possible risk of intussusception, which is a treatable condition when promptly detected. CDC continues to recommend routine rotavirus vaccination of US infants.

Studies in other countries have also found increased risk for intussusception associated with the 2 vaccines, but the results have been variable.[39–42] The WHO has upheld its recommendation for universal rotavirus vaccination because the substantial benefits of vaccination to prevent hospitalizations and death far outweigh the potential low-level risk of intussusception.[33,43]

Rotavirus Vaccine Coverage

United States
The National Immunization Survey is a large, on-going survey of immunization coverage among US preschool children 19 through 35 months old. The most recent data showing national vaccination coverage rates for children born January 2010 to May 2012 was published in August 2014.[44] The survey showed coverage increased from 2012 to 2013 for a complete series of rotavirus vaccine from 68.6% to 72.6%.

Global
WHO and UNICEF estimate national and global infant immunization coverage yearly based on administrative data received from each country. The latest WHO data for global coverage is from 2013 and shows that rotavirus vaccine was introduced in 52 countries, up from 41 in 2012. Global coverage was estimated at 14% with most rotavirus vaccine usage in high- and middle-income countries.

Rotavirus Surveillance to Monitor Vaccine Programs

United States surveillance programs

Rotavirus gastroenteritis is not a reportable disease in the United States, and testing for rotavirus infection is not often performed when a child seeks medical care for gastroenteritis. Methods of surveillance for rotavirus disease at the national level include review of national hospital discharge databases for rotavirus-specific or rotavirus-compatible diagnoses, surveillance for rotavirus disease at 3 sites that participate in the New Vaccine Surveillance Network, and reports of rotavirus detection from CDC National Respiratory and Enteric Virus Surveillance System (NREVSS).

The CDC has established a national strain surveillance system of sentinel laboratories to monitor circulating rotavirus strains before and after the introduction of rotavirus vaccine. This system is designed to detect new or unusual strains causing gastroenteritis that might not be prevented effectively by vaccination, which might affect the success of the vaccination program.

World Health Organization surveillance programs

Since 2008, the WHO has coordinated the Global Rotavirus Surveillance Network, a network of sentinel surveillance hospitals and laboratories that report to ministries of health and WHO clinical features and rotavirus testing data for children aged less than 5 years hospitalized with acute gastroenteritis.[45] As of 2012, the Global Rotavirus Surveillance Network included 178 sentinel surveillance sites in 60 countries.

Evaluation of the Effect of Rotavirus Vaccine Programs

As rotavirus vaccination programs are implemented, it is important to evaluate the effect of vaccine on rotavirus disease and epidemiology for several reasons (**Box 5**).[46]

The Effectiveness of Rotavirus Vaccination in the Prevention of Rotavirus Disease

Unlike efficacy studies that are conducted in a carefully controlled setting, studies on vaccine effectiveness compare the risks of disease outcomes in vaccinated or non-vaccinated populations in a real-life setting. Since the introduction of rotavirus vaccines into national immunization programs beginning in 2006, studies have been

---

Box 5
Rationale for evaluation of the effect of rotavirus vaccine programs

First, routine immunization occurs in conditions different from the ideal clinical trial setting. Monitoring after-licensure effectiveness of rotavirus vaccine is important to assure that the expected benefits of rotavirus vaccine programs are achieved.

Second, assessing protection in infants through the first and second years of life is crucial for the success of a rotavirus vaccination program because infancy is when most severe disease and mortality from rotavirus occur.

Third, assessing whether vaccination results in herd immunity is important because a vaccine with indirect protection could provide substantially greater benefits than expected on the basis of direct efficacy.

Fourth, changes in the epidemiology of rotavirus disease may occur after licensure, such as duration of protection, changes in age-specific and seasonal incidence of disease, and timing of epidemics. These changes may be important in immunization program planning.

Fifth, surveillance is important to describe serotype distributions in individual countries and worldwide to identify newly emerging strains or changes in strain distribution because these may compromise the effectiveness of rotavirus vaccines.

conducted to assess vaccine effectiveness in a variety of low-, low-middle-, middle-, and high-income countries. The real-world effectiveness data for both vaccines are consistent with efficacy data obtained from clinical trials. In high-income countries such as the United States,[47] Australia,[48] Austria,[49] and Israel,[50] vaccine effectiveness was similar to estimates from the clinical trials (>85%). In the upper-middle income Latin American countries of Mexico and Brazil, effectiveness estimates have ranged from 79% to 94%, and in the lower middle income country of El Salvador, effectiveness was estimated at 76%.[51–54] Notably, the lowest effectiveness (46%–64%) was observed in Nicaragua and Malawi, the most impoverished settings where vaccine performance in routine use has been evaluated to date.[55–57]

In a review of data from the first 7 years of vaccine use in the United States, both recommended rotavirus vaccines, RV5 and RV1, have been shown to be highly effective in preventing outcomes of severe disease in a variety of settings.[47] Vaccine effectiveness ranged from 84% to 100% for RV5 and 70% to 91% for RV1.

Duration of Immunity

In high-income countries, rotavirus vaccines have been shown to protect infants through the third year of life.[58,59] In low-income countries, the rotavirus threat is greatest during the first year of life. In clinical studies in Africa and Asia, rotavirus vaccines have been shown to provide the greatest protection during this first year.[28–30] Efficacy in the second year of life may be lower in low-income countries, but further evaluation is required to understand in which populations and under what circumstances vaccine efficacy declines.[21,28–30,60]

The Impact of Rotavirus Vaccination on the Health Burden of Rotavirus Disease

Rapid and significant declines in hospitalizations and deaths due to rotavirus and all-cause diarrhea have been observed in many of the countries that have introduced rotavirus vaccines into their national immunization programs, including Austria, Australia, Belgium, Bolivia, Brazil, El Salvador, Finland, Honduras, Mexico, Nicaragua, Panama, Taiwan, the United States, and Venezuela.[61]

A review of the impact of rotavirus vaccines after 7 years of vaccine use in the United States found sustained decreases in the burden of rotavirus disease in a variety of settings ranging from the local to the national level.[47] A recent review of available data from countries routinely using rotavirus vaccines in their national immunization programs found that rotavirus vaccines have reduced rotavirus hospitalizations by 49% to 92% and all-cause diarrhea hospitalizations by 17% to 55%.[62] In addition, the review found that all-cause diarrhea deaths were reduced by 22% to 50% in some settings.[62]

Studies comparing the numbers or proportions of rotavirus-positive tests before and after introduction of the rotavirus vaccination program are useful in evaluating vaccine impact. Sentinel laboratory surveillance from the CDC NREVSS has demonstrated a decline in the number of rotavirus-positive tests in the United States as well as the total number of tests performed compared with the prevaccine years (2000–2006).[63] During 7 postvaccine years (2007–2014), the peak rotavirus positivity rates ranged from 10.9% to 27.3% compared with 43.1% in the 7 prevaccine years combined (**Fig. 1**).

Herd Immunity After Rotavirus Vaccination

Herd immunity occurs as a result of decreased transmission of rotavirus in the community and provides indirect protection to unvaccinated individuals. The rotavirus vaccination schedule should be completed by 32 weeks of age in the United States

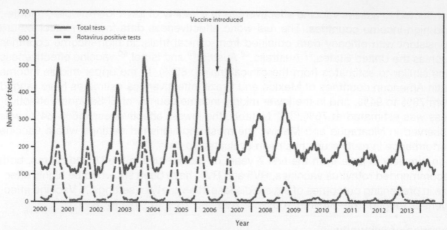

Fig. 1. Total and positive rotavirus tests, NREVSS data—United States, 2000–2014. (*From* Aliabadi N, Tate JE, Haynes AK, et al; Centers for Disease Control and Prevention. Sustained decrease in laboratory detection of rotavirus after implementation of routine vaccination— United States, 2000–2014. MMWR Morb Mortal Wkly Rep 2015;64(13):342.)

and by 26 weeks in Europe. There have been no catch-up vaccination programs in older children. In some countries where rotavirus vaccines have been introduced, significant reductions in rotavirus diarrhea hospitalizations in unvaccinated adults and children have been seen, suggesting rotavirus vaccines provide indirect protection to unvaccinated children and adults by reducing spread of the virus.[64–68] This finding is important because herd immunity will be important in resource-poor countries where vaccine efficacy and coverage tend to be lower.

Changing Epidemiology and Seasonality of Rotavirus Disease After Vaccine Introduction

In the United States, there were alterations in the rotavirus season following the introduction of rotavirus vaccine. Analysis of data from the NRVESS shows postvaccine rotavirus seasons with later onset and shorter duration (**Fig. 2**), a biennial pattern of rotavirus activity emerged in the postvaccine era, with years of low activity and highly erratic seasonality alternating with years of greater activity, and seasonality similar to those in the prevaccine era.[63] Studies from Belgium also show a shift in the onset of the epidemic by 1 to 2 months has occurred after rotavirus vaccination.[69]

Effect of Vaccination on Rotavirus Strain Circulation and Emergence

Rotavirus vaccines need to provide cross-protection against multiple rotavirus serotypes because circulating strains vary and multiple strains can circulate within the same region at the same time. Concerns exist about whether monovalent (RV1) and pentavalent (RV5) rotavirus vaccines provide adequate protection against diverse strains and whether vaccine introduction will lead to selective pressure. Multiple studies have found that vaccine introduction has not led to significant strain shifts or escape mutants as yet.

A systematic review of published studies investigated the distribution of rotavirus strains and strain-specific rotavirus vaccine effectiveness after vaccine introduction (**Table 4**).[70] No difference was noted in vaccine effectiveness for either RV1 or RV5 in any setting. Prevalent strains in countries using RV1 were G2P[4] (50%)

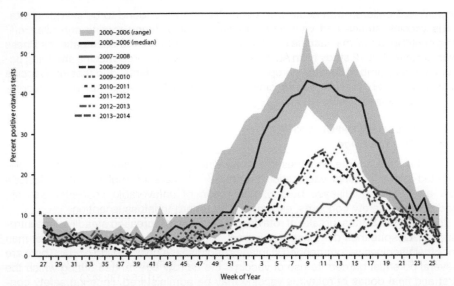

Fig. 2. Rotavirus season duration and peak activity by reporting years (prevaccine 2000–2006 and postvaccine 2007–2011), NREVSS data—United States, 2000–2014. [a] Dashed line indicates the 10% threshold of numbers of positive test results, which is used to determine onset and offset of a rotavirus season. (*From* Aliabadi N, Tate JE, Haynes AK, et al; Centers for Disease Control and Prevention. Sustained decrease in laboratory detection of rotavirus after implementation of routine vaccination—United States, 2000–2014. MMWR Morb Mortal Wkly Rep 2015;64(13):340.)

and G1P[8] (22%), and those in countries using RV5 were G1P[8] (33%) and G2P[4] (30%). Sustained predominance of a single strain was not recorded. The authors concluded RV1 and RV5 are equally effective against homotypic and heterotypic rotavirus strains.

A final concern comes from the ability of rotavirus to undergo reassortment with wild-type or vaccine-derived strains. Little is known about the frequency with which reassortment occurs or the resulting clinical outcome. A 2012 report from Texas

Table 4
Strain-specific rotavirus vaccine effectiveness

| | Pooled Vaccine Effectiveness | |
Setting	RV1	RV5
High-income countries	94% against homotypic strains	83% against homotypic strains
	71% against partly heterotypic strains	82% against single-antigen vaccine type strains
	87% against fully heterotypic strains	82% against partly heterotypic strains
		75% against single-antigen nonvaccine type strains
Middle-income countries	59% against homotypic strains	70% against single-antigen vaccine type strains
	72% against partly heterotypic strains	37% against partly heterotypic strains
	47% against fully heterotypic strains	87% against single-antigen nonvaccine type strains

describes 5 children with acute gastroenteritis who were found to be shedding rotavirus vaccine strains and vaccine-reassortant strains during routine surveillance.[71] The contribution of the vaccine or vaccine-reassortant strain to each patient's illness was unclear. A 2012 study from Australia suggests that rotavirus vaccine shedding occurs naturally among a sizable proportion of vaccinated infants, and that intravaccine reassortant events resulting in vaccine-associated gastroenteritis may be more common than originally believed.[72]

CHALLENGES AND OPPORTUNITIES
Low Vaccine Coverage

There are high-income countries in Europe where rotavirus vaccines are not implemented in the national vaccination program.[73] Barriers to implementation include low awareness of disease burden, perception of unfavorable cost-effectiveness, and potential safety concerns, especially with regard to intussusception.

In the United States, uptake of rotavirus vaccines has increased steadily since introduction. Despite their demonstrated impact, rotavirus vaccine coverage is lower than for other vaccines recommended in infancy and disease continues to occur. There are several potential barriers to use of vaccine: the narrow age ranges during which the first and final doses of rotavirus vaccine may be administered, lingering safety concerns related to intussusception, hesitancy about use of a new live-attenuated oral vaccine, and issues regarding vaccine cost and insurance reimbursement. A recent study observed the highest detection of rotavirus disease among locations with low rotavirus vaccine coverage, suggesting that ongoing disease transmission is related to failure to vaccinate.[74] The authors concluded that educational efforts focusing on timely rotavirus vaccine administration to age eligible infants are needed.

The GAVI Alliance, a global health partnership that works to increase access to vaccines, is supporting the introduction of rotavirus vaccines in some of the world's poorest countries. As of April 2015, thirty-five countries have introduced rotavirus vaccines with GAVI's support, but vaccine still remains out of reach for many in the developing world.

In GAVI-eligible countries, where 95% of deaths due to rotavirus occur, more than 2.4 million child deaths can be prevented by 2030 by accelerating access to lifesaving rotavirus vaccines.[75] If used in all GAVI-eligible countries, rotavirus vaccines could prevent an estimated 180,000 deaths[75] and avert 6 million clinic and hospital visits each year, thereby saving US$68 million annually in treatment costs.[75]

Need for Large Field Efficacy Trials and After-Licensure Surveillance for New Vaccine Candidates

Without correlates of immunity, each new rotavirus vaccine candidate will require large field trials to demonstrate efficacy. Although a placebo control study is the preferred scientific way to conduct such trials, the availability of the 2 currently licensed vaccines limits the ethical justification of conducting placebo control studies. In addition, the early experience with RRV-TV and intussusception means that substantial aftermarketing surveillance activities need to be put into place in every country where rotavirus vaccines are introduced to identify this condition and its possible association with vaccination.

Diminished Efficacy in High-Burden Low-Income Settings

Clinical studies of the currently licensed oral, live rotavirus vaccines have found that (as with other oral, live vaccines) performance was diminished in high-burden, low-income settings. This diminished performance may be due to elevated maternal antibodies, potential interference by other oral vaccines, and coinfections of the digestive tract. The development of new, more affordable and potentially more effective rotavirus vaccines could make an enormous impact on public health by reducing rotavirus-related illness and deaths worldwide, particularly in low-resource countries.

Need for Long-Term Surveillance to Monitor the Effects of Vaccination Programs

Long-term monitoring will need to continue to assess the effects of rotavirus immunization programs, and epidemiologic strain surveillance is necessary to determine whether changes in strain ecology will affect the rotavirus vaccine effectiveness and whether rotaviruses with the ability to evade vaccine immunity emerge. Expansion of rotavirus surveillance efforts to low-income countries will be crucial to identify emergence of new strains and to assess strain-specific vaccine effectiveness in this setting. Continued surveillance will be necessary to assess the rate of occurrence and clinical relevance of vaccine strains and vaccine-reassortant strains in symptomatic and asymptomatic pediatric rotavirus infections.

Research Needs

Research is needed to define the impact of factors such as malnutrition, aberrant intestinal microflora, concomitant infections, and pre-existing immunity as well as of host genetic factors on the immunogenicity of rotavirus vaccines.

The need for more efficacious vaccines is being addressed by research into novel approaches for rotavirus vaccine development. Because live virus vaccines have potential inadequacies, such as side effects due to insufficient attenuation, adverse reactions associated with viral replication, or insufficient efficacies against rotavirus disease, non-living rotavirus vaccine candidates are being developed. Currently, 3 types of candidates are in development: viruslike particles, recombinant VP6 proteins, and inactivated rotaviruses. These novel approaches are being pursued in preclinical and clinical studies.

REFERENCES

1. Tate JE, Burton AH, Boschi-Pinto C, et al. 2008 estimate of worldwide rotavirus-associated mortality in children younger than 5 years before the introduction of universal rotavirus vaccination programmes: a systematic review and meta-analysis. Lancet Infect Dis 2012;12(2):136–41.
2. Glass RI, Bresee J, Jiang B, et al. Rotavirus and rotavirus vaccines. Adv Exp Med Biol 2006;582:45–54.
3. Rotavirus surveillance worldwide - 2009. Wkly Epidemiol Rec 2011;86(18):174–6 [in English, French].
4. Kotloff KL, Nataro JP, Blackwelder WC, et al. Burden and aetiology of diarrhoeal disease in infants and young children in developing countries (the Global Enteric Multicenter Study, GEMS): a prospective, case-control study. Lancet 2013; 382(9888):209–22.
5. Malek MA, Curns AT, Holman RC, et al. Diarrhea- and rotavirus-associated hospitalizations among children less than 5 years of age: United states, 1997 and 2000. Pediatrics 2006;117(6):1887–92.
6. Fischer TK, Viboud C, Parashar U, et al. Hospitalizations and deaths from diarrhea and rotavirus among children <5 years of age in the United States, 1993-2003. J Infect Dis 2007;195(8):1117–25.

7. Cortese MM, Parashar UD. Prevention of rotavirus gastroenteritis among infants and children: recommendations of the Advisory Committee on Immunization Practices (ACIP). MMWR Recomm Rep 2009;58(RR-2):1–25.
8. Coffin SE, Elser J, Marchant C, et al. Impact of acute rotavirus gastroenteritis on pediatric outpatient practices in the United States. Pediatr Infect Dis J 2006; 25(7):584–9.
9. Widdowson MA, Meltzer MI, Zhang X, et al. Cost-effectiveness and potential impact of rotavirus vaccination in the United States. Pediatrics 2007;119(4): 684–97.
10. Staat MA, Azimi PH, Berke T, et al. Clinical presentations of rotavirus infection among hospitalized children. Pediatr Infect Dis J 2002;21(3):221–7.
11. Banyai K, Laszlo B, Duque J, et al. Systematic review of regional and temporal trends in global rotavirus strain diversity in the pre rotavirus vaccine era: insights for understanding the impact of rotavirus vaccination programs. Vaccine 2012; 30(Suppl 1):A122–30.
12. Fu C, He Q, Xu J, et al. Effectiveness of the Lanzhou lamb rotavirus vaccine against gastroenteritis among children. Vaccine 2012;31(1):154–8.
13. Rennels MB, Glass RI, Dennehy PH, et al. Safety and efficacy of high-dose rhesus-human reassortant rotavirus vaccines–report of the national multicenter trial. United States rotavirus vaccine efficacy group. Pediatrics 1996;97(1):7–13.
14. Rotavirus vaccine for the prevention of rotavirus gastroenteritis among children. Recommendations of the Advisory Committee on Immunization Practices (ACIP). MMWR Recomm Rep 1999;48(RR-2):1–20.
15. Centers for Disease Control and Prevention (CDC). Intussusception among recipients of rotavirus vaccine–United States, 1998-1999. MMWR Morb Mortal Wkly Rep 1999;48(27):577–81.
16. Murphy TV, Gargiullo PM, Massoudi MS, et al. Intussusception among infants given an oral rotavirus vaccine. N Engl J Med 2001;344(8):564–72.
17. Peter G, Myers MG. Intussusception, rotavirus, and oral vaccines: summary of a workshop. Pediatrics 2002;110(6):e67.
18. Centers for Disease Control and Prevention (CDC). Withdrawal of rotavirus vaccine recommendation. MMWR Morb Mortal Wkly Rep 1999;48(43):1007.
19. Vesikari T, Matson DO, Dennehy P, et al. Safety and efficacy of a pentavalent human-bovine (WC3) reassortant rotavirus vaccine. N Engl J Med 2006;354(1): 23–33.
20. Block SL, Vesikari T, Goveia MG, et al. Efficacy, immunogenicity, and safety of a pentavalent human-bovine (WC3) reassortant rotavirus vaccine at the end of shelf life. Pediatrics 2007;119(1):11–8.
21. Bhandari N, Rongsen-Chandola T, Bavdekar A, et al. Efficacy of a monovalent human-bovine (116E) rotavirus vaccine in Indian children in the second year of life. Vaccine 2014;32(Suppl 1):A110–6.
22. Bhandari N, Rongsen-Chandola T, Bavdekar A, et al. Efficacy of a monovalent human-bovine (116E) rotavirus vaccine in Indian infants: a randomised, double-blind, placebo-controlled trial. Lancet 2014;383(9935):2136–43.
23. Bernstein DI, Ward RL. Rotarix: development of a live attenuated monovalent human rotavirus vaccine. Pediatr Ann 2006;35(1):38–43.
24. Ruiz-Palacios GM, Perez-Schael I, Velazquez FR, et al. Safety and efficacy of an attenuated vaccine against severe rotavirus gastroenteritis. N Engl J Med 2006; 354(1):11–22.
25. Vesikari T, Karvonen A, Prymula R, et al. Efficacy of human rotavirus vaccine against rotavirus gastroenteritis during the first 2 years of life in European

infants: randomised, double-blind controlled study. Lancet 2007;370(9601): 1757–63.

26. Linhares AC, Velazquez FR, Perez-Schael I, et al. Efficacy and safety of an oral live attenuated human rotavirus vaccine against rotavirus gastroenteritis during the first 2 years of life in Latin American infants: a randomised, double-blind, placebo-controlled phase III study. Lancet 2008;371(9619):1181–9.

27. Vesikari T, Itzler R, Karvonen A, et al. RotaTeq, a pentavalent rotavirus vaccine: efficacy and safety among infants in Europe. Vaccine 2009;28(2):345–51.

28. Armah GE, Sow SO, Breiman RF, et al. Efficacy of pentavalent rotavirus vaccine against severe rotavirus gastroenteritis in infants in developing countries in sub-Saharan Africa: a randomised, double-blind, placebo-controlled trial. Lancet 2010;376(9741):606–14.

29. Madhi SA, Cunliffe NA, Steele D, et al. Effect of human rotavirus vaccine on severe diarrhea in African infants. N Engl J Med 2010;362(4):289–98.

30. Zaman K, Dang DA, Victor JC, et al. Efficacy of pentavalent rotavirus vaccine against severe rotavirus gastroenteritis in infants in developing countries in Asia: a randomised, double-blind, placebo-controlled trial. Lancet 2010;376(9741):615–23.

31. Soares-Weiser K, Maclehose H, Bergman H, et al. Vaccines for preventing rotavirus diarrhoea: vaccines in use. Cochrane Database Syst Rev 2012;(11):CD008521.

32. World Health Organization. Rotavirus vaccines: an update. Wkly Epidemiol Rec 2009;84(50):533–40 [in English, French].

33. Rotavirus vaccines. WHO position paper - January 2013. Wkly Epidemiol Rec 2013;88(5):49–64 [in English, French].

34. Committee on Infectious Diseases of the American Academy of Pediatrics. Prevention of rotavirus disease: updated guidelines for use of rotavirus vaccine. Pediatrics 2009;123(5):1412–20.

35. Shui IM, Baggs J, Patel M, et al. Risk of intussusception following administration of a pentavalent rotavirus vaccine in us infants. JAMA 2012;307(6):598–604.

36. Loughlin J, Mast TC, Doherty M, et al. Postmarketing evaluation of the short-term safety of the pentavalent rotavirus vaccine. Pediatr Infect Dis J 2012;31(3):292–6.

37. Yen C, Tate JE, Steiner CA, et al. Trends in intussusception hospitalizations among US infants before and after implementation of the rotavirus vaccination program, 2000-2009. J Infect Dis 2012;206(1):41–8.

38. Desai R, Cortese MM, Meltzer MI, et al. Potential intussusception risk versus benefits of rotavirus vaccination in the United States. Pediatr Infect Dis J 2013;32(1):1–7.

39. Buttery JP, Danchin MH, Lee KJ, et al. Intussusception following rotavirus vaccine administration: post-marketing surveillance in the national immunization program in Australia. Vaccine 2011;29(16):3061–6.

40. Patel MM, Lopez-Collada VR, Bulhoes MM, et al. Intussusception risk and health benefits of rotavirus vaccination in Mexico and Brazil. N Engl J Med 2011; 364(24):2283–92.

41. Velazquez FR, Colindres RE, Grajales C, et al. Postmarketing surveillance of intussusception following mass introduction of the attenuated human rotavirus vaccine in Mexico. Pediatr Infect Dis J 2012;31(7):736–44.

42. Carlin JB, Macartney KK, Lee KJ, et al. Intussusception risk and disease prevention associated with rotavirus vaccines in Australia's National Immunization Program. Clin Infect Dis 2013;57(10):1427–34.

43. Global Advisory Committee on Vaccine Safety, 11-12 June 2014. Wkly Epidemiol Rec 2014;89(29):325–35 [in English, French].

44. Elam-Evans LD, Yankey D, Singleton JA, et al, Centers for Disease Control and Prevention. National, state, and selected local area vaccination coverage among children aged 19-35 months - United States, 2013. MMWR Morb Mortal Wkly Rep 2014;63(34):741–8.

45. Agocs MM, Serhan F, Yen C, et al. Who global rotavirus surveillance network: a strategic review of the first 5 years, 2008-2012. MMWR Morb Mortal Wkly Rep 2014;63(29):634–7.

46. Patel MM, Steele D, Gentsch JR, et al. Real-world impact of rotavirus vaccination. Pediatr Infect Dis J 2011;30(1 Suppl):S1–5.

47. Rha B, Tate JE, Payne DC, et al. Effectiveness and impact of rotavirus vaccines in the United States - 2006-2012. Expert Rev Vaccines 2014;13(3):365–76.

48. Buttery JP, Lambert SB, Grimwood K, et al. Reduction in rotavirus-associated acute gastroenteritis following introduction of rotavirus vaccine into Australia's national childhood vaccine schedule. Pediatr Infect Dis J 2011;30(1 Suppl):S25–9.

49. Paulke-Korinek M, Rendi-Wagner P, Kundi M, et al. Universal mass vaccination against rotavirus gastroenteritis: impact on hospitalization rates in Austrian children. Pediatr Infect Dis J 2010;29(4):319–23.

50. Muhsen K, Shulman L, Kasem E, et al. Effectiveness of rotavirus vaccines for prevention of rotavirus gastroenteritis-associated hospitalizations in Israel: a case-control study. Hum Vaccin 2010;6(6):450–4.

51. Correia JB, Patel MM, Nakagomi O, et al. Effectiveness of monovalent rotavirus vaccine (Rotarix) against severe diarrhea caused by serotypically unrelated G2P[4] strains in Brazil. J Infect Dis 2010;201(3):363–9.

52. Gurgel RQ, Correia JB, Cuevas LE. Effect of rotavirus vaccination on circulating virus strains. Lancet 2008;371(9609):301–2.

53. Justino MC, Linhares AC, Lanzieri TM, et al. Effectiveness of the monovalent G1P [8] human rotavirus vaccine against hospitalization for severe G2P[4] rotavirus gastroenteritis in Belem, Brazil. Pediatr Infect Dis J 2011;30(5):396–401.

54. Yen C, Figueroa JR, Uribe ES, et al. Monovalent rotavirus vaccine provides protection against an emerging fully heterotypic G9P[4] rotavirus strain in Mexico. J Infect Dis 2011;204(5):783–6.

55. Mast TC, Khawaja S, Espinoza F, et al. Case-control study of the effectiveness of vaccination with pentavalent rotavirus vaccine in Nicaragua. Pediatr Infect Dis J 2011;30(11):e209–15.

56. Patel M, Pedreira C, De Oliveira LH, et al. Association between pentavalent rotavirus vaccine and severe rotavirus diarrhea among children in Nicaragua. JAMA 2009;301(21):2243–51.

57. Bar-Zeev N, Kapanda L, Tate JE, et al. Effectiveness of a monovalent rotavirus vaccine in infants in Malawi after programmatic roll-out: an observational and case-control study. Lancet Infect Dis 2015;15(4):422–8.

58. Boom JA, Tate JE, Sahni LC, et al. Sustained protection from pentavalent rotavirus vaccination during the second year of life at a large, urban United States pediatric hospital. Pediatr Infect Dis J 2010;29(12):1133–5.

59. Vesikari T, Karvonen A, Ferrante SA, et al. Sustained efficacy of the pentavalent rotavirus vaccine, RV5, up to 3.1 years following the last dose of vaccine. Pediatr Infect Dis J 2010;29(10):957–63.

60. Neuzil KM, Zaman K, Victor JC. A proposed framework for evaluating and comparing efficacy estimates in clinical trials of new rotavirus vaccines. Vaccine 2014;32(Suppl 1):A179–84.

61. Rotavirus vaccine impact data. Available at: http://sites.path.org/rotavirusvaccine/vaccine-impact-data/. Accessed April 6, 2015.

62. Tate JE, Parashar UD. Rotavirus vaccines in routine use. Clin Infect Dis 2014; 59(9):1291–301.
63. Aliabadi N, Tate JE, Haynes AK, et al, Centers for Disease Control and Prevention. Sustained decrease in laboratory detection of rotavirus after implementation of routine vaccination—United States, 2000-2014. MMWR Morb Mortal Wkly Rep 2015;64(13):337–42.
64. Lopman BA, Curns AT, Yen C, et al. Infant rotavirus vaccination may provide indirect protection to older children and adults in the United States. J Infect Dis 2011;204(7):980–6.
65. Anderson EJ, Shippee DB, Weinrobe MH, et al. Indirect protection of adults from rotavirus by pediatric rotavirus vaccination. Clin Infect Dis 2013;56(6):755–60.
66. Paulke-Korinek M, Kundi M, Rendi-Wagner P, et al. Herd immunity after two years of the universal mass vaccination program against rotavirus gastroenteritis in Austria. Vaccine 2011;29(15):2791–6.
67. Cortese MM, Dahl RM, Curns AT, et al. Protection against gastroenteritis in US households with children who received rotavirus vaccine. J Infect Dis 2015; 211(4):558–62.
68. Gastanaduy PA, Curns AT, Parashar UD, et al. Gastroenteritis hospitalizations in older children and adults in the United States before and after implementation of infant rotavirus vaccination. JAMA 2013;310(8):851–3.
69. Braeckman T, Van Herck K, Raes M, et al. Rotavirus vaccines in Belgium: policy and impact. Pediatr Infect Dis J 2011;30(1 Suppl):S21–4.
70. Leshem E, Lopman B, Glass R, et al. Distribution of rotavirus strains and strain-specific effectiveness of the rotavirus vaccine after its introduction: a systematic review and meta-analysis. Lancet Infect Dis 2014;14(9):847–56.
71. Boom JA, Sahni LC, Payne DC, et al. Symptomatic infection and detection of vaccine and vaccine-reassortant rotavirus strains in 5 children: a case series. J Infect Dis 2012;206(8):1275–9.
72. Donato CM, Ch'ng LS, Boniface KF, et al. Identification of strains of Rota Teq rotavirus vaccine in infants with gastroenteritis following routine vaccination. J Infect Dis 2012;206(3):377–83.
73. Parez N, Giaquinto C, Du Roure C, et al. Rotavirus vaccination in Europe: drivers and barriers. Lancet Infect Dis 2014;14(5):416–25.
74. Sahni LC, Tate JE, Payne DC, et al. Variation in rotavirus vaccine coverage by provider location and subsequent disease burden. Pediatrics 2015;135(2): e432–9.
75. Atherly DE, Lewis KD, Tate J, et al. Projected health and economic impact of rotavirus vaccination in GAVI-eligible countries: 2011–2030. Vaccine 2012;30(Suppl 1):A7–14.
76. Franco MA, Angel J, Greenberg HB. Immunity and correlates of protection for rotavirus vaccines. Vaccine 2006;24(15):2718–31.
77. Velazquez FR, Matson DO, Calva JJ, et al. Rotavirus infections in infants as protection against subsequent infections. N Engl J Med 1996;335(14):1022–8.

Rabies
Rare Human Infection – Common Questions

Rodney E. Willoughby Jr, MD

KEYWORDS

- Rabies • Lyssavirus • Encephalitis • Diagnosis • Therapy • Mortality
- Brain diseases • Biopterin

KEY POINTS

- Rabies may cause a continuum of disease severity and is treatable.
- Modern pre-exposure prophylaxis and postexposure prophylaxis (PEP) is highly effective.
- Rabies behaves like and is treated as an acquired metabolic disorder.

Rabies is an acute and rapidly progressive encephalitis that is almost always fatal. It is a syndrome caused by 12 lyssavirus species, including rabies virus (genotype 1 lyssavirus). Rabies is a global zoonosis – only the continent of Antarctica is rabies-free. Rabies virus is the only lyssavirus present in the Americas. Many so-called rabies-free countries contain other lyssaviruses in wildlife, but the intersection of the reservoir species for these lyssaviruses with humans is rare.

NATURAL HISTORY

Lyssaviruses are negative-sense, single-stranded, enveloped RNA viruses that contain a single-surface glycoprotein and a ribonucleoprotein core. Rabies virus is transmitted by saliva or infected neural tissue. It is rapidly inactivated by desiccation and sunlight. Infection requires contamination of infected saliva or neural tissue into a bite wound or broken skin or onto mucosa. Natural transmission by aerosol is debated. Ingestion requires large doses for infection. There is no hematogenous or congenital transmission. Blood, urine, and feces are not infectious in animals or humans. There have been 4 outbreaks of rabies associated with solid organ transplantation and 13 by corneal implantation. Rabies virus is considered a potential biological weapon.

The author has nothing to disclose.
Pediatric Infectious Diseases, Children's Hospital of Wisconsin, C450, PO Box 1997, Milwaukee, WI 53201-1997, USA
E-mail address: rewillou@mcw.edu

Infect Dis Clin N Am 29 (2015) 637–650
http://dx.doi.org/10.1016/j.idc.2015.07.006
0891-5520/15/$ – see front matter © 2015 Elsevier Inc. All rights reserved.

id.theclinics.com

Rabies virus replicates poorly and at low levels in local tissues, including muscle (dog rabies) and skin (bat rabies). Inefficient virus replication avoids immune detection and results in highly variable and often prolonged incubation periods (up to 7 years).[1] There is no known mechanism for latent infection by rabies virus, although the incubation period is prolonged during hibernation. Louis Pasteur capitalized on the long incubation period of rabies to develop highly effective PEP. Rabies virus is highly neurotropic, replicating rapidly once it enters neurons. Because the nervous system is a privileged immunologic site, rabies virus continues to evade the adaptive immune response for many days after entering the central nervous system (CNS). Motor fibers transmit rabies virus efficiently by rapid retrograde axonal transport and it is disseminated exclusively across synapses, at the rate of approximtely 1 synaptic network every 12 hours. Dorsal root ganglia are also infected by rabies virus and contribute to the clinical syndrome but do not extend the infection.[2] Synaptic transmission within the brain and spinal cord to autonomic nerves results in prominent clinical signs that lag behind motor and sensory findings.[2]

The mechanism of death from rabies remains unclear. The virus is poorly cytopathic and poorly immunogenic, so anatomic damage is minimal. Behavioral effects are initially subtle and remain intermittent until the patient lapses into coma within a week of hospitalization. In animal models, there are several days during which the CNS is massively infected, yet there are no symptoms or signs. Once in the CNS, the virus engages in centrifugal spread, involving all peripheral nerves. The peripheral spread to the salivary glands and the subtle, intermittent behavioral changes facilitate transmission to the next host. Dysautonomia, sensory denervation, and paralysis ensue. Humans and most small rodents and lagomorphs are dead-end hosts. There has never been a proven case of human-to-human transmission of rabies through clinical care or at autopsy, other than by solid organ or corneal transplantation.[3]

The clinical prodrome is vague, variable in duration (3–10 days) and flulike, often with sore throat and sleep disturbance. This is followed by episodic changes in alertness, agitation, aggression, panic, and hallucinations. Characteristic features that assist in distinguishing rabies from other forms of encephalitis and encephalopathy are listed in **Box 1**. Although classic teaching differentiates "furious" (encephalitic) and "dumb" (paralytic) rabies, in my experience there tends to be a continuum of signs and symptoms. Paresis occurs in both. A case report and a dog model suggest that

---

Box 1
Distinguishing characteristics of rabies encephalitis

1. Episodes of altered arousal, behavior, cognition, and dysautonomia interspersed with complete normalcy

2. Pain, pruritus, and dysesthesias referable to the bitten limb

3. Myoclonic jerks, paresis referable to the bitten limb

4. Dysphagia, hydrophobia, and aerophobia

5. Dysautonomia, including catecholamine surges, bradyarrhythmias, hypersalivation, piloerection, sweating, and priapism.

6. Guillain-Barré–like syndromes that include urinary and fecal retention or other dysautonomia

7. Orofacial dyskinesias and myokymia

8. History of exposure (foreign travel, immigration, attic remodeling, cabin ownership, hunting or dressing the game, spelunking, wildlife rehabilitation or organ transplantation)

the immune response to the rabies virus may convert encephalitic rabies to the paralytic form,[4,5] which is similar in pathogenesis to animal models of abortive rabies.[6,7]

Rabies is rapidly progressive, with most patients in endemic areas dying within 3 days of hospitalization and without detectable antibody. Autopsy after early demise shows minimal findings of perivenular inflammation and occasional viral inclusions (Negri bodies) in the hippocampus and cerebellum. There is little apoptosis or necrosis of neurons. With modern critical care, median survival is 18 days. Autopsies done in the second week, after rabies antibody is detected, show heterogeneous clearance of the rabies virus peripherally and in the CNS. Cultivable virus clears first, followed by spatial dissociation of rabies virus nucleoprotein and genome.[6,8–10] Histology and neuroimaging are reflective of the medical complications leading to demise.

There are rare individuals who fulfill diagnostic criteria for rabies yet have milder disease, suggesting that there might be a continuum of disease caused by lyssaviruses.[11–13] The continuum of rabies disease is well described in animal models of rabies, notably using attenuated viruses and genetically altered hosts.[14] There are also provocative serologic studies in high-risk populations suggesting seroconversion of individuals without known clinical disease.[15–18] This should not be possible if rabies is uniformly fatal. In some subjects, there was no detection of neutralizing antibody despite antibodies to the ribonucleoprotein.[11,15,19] Whether these persons truly had rabies is controversial.

DIAGNOSIS

There are 2 diagnostic steps to be reviewed. The first is diagnosis of exposure to rabies, to determine the need for PEP. The second is the diagnosis of rabies, which is important to limit care or engage in intensive care of rabies and for infection control.

Rabies exposure is determined by the bite of a potentially rabies virus-infected animal. In most of the world, the cosmopolitan strain of dog rabies is transmitted by dog or cat bite. I have cared for several patients who were infected with the rabies virus by the licks of puppies to the hands, feet, or ankles. Cats transmit more rabies than dogs in the United States and can also transmit bat, raccoon, skunk, fox, or other phylogenies of rabies virus through their hunting behavior.[20] Bats carry a different phylogeny of rabies virus and, outside of the Americas, carry other lyssaviruses as well. Bat teeth are very small and bites can be difficult to sense or find by examination. In the United States, almost all rabies is bat-associated and in 78% of victims, there is no history of animal exposure.[21] When a bat exposure was documented, it always involved physical contact with the bat. The lack of regular history of bat exposure among rabies fatalities in the United States led to epidemiologic criteria for exposure to rabies requiring prophylaxis based on proximity to the bat and the quality of the historian (**Table 1**).[22] These criteria were challenged on economic grounds.[23]

The diagnosis of incubating rabies cannot be made. The virus replicates at low levels and most patients with rabies die without detectable immune response. On the other hand, PEP remains effective until just days before symptoms develop.

Delayed diagnosis of rabies is common; 38% of rabies cases in the United States are diagnosed at autopsy.[21] The diagnosis of rabies requires a compatible acute neurologic syndrome and confirmatory laboratory tests because there are many mimics of human rabies (**Box 2**). Hydrophobia and aerophobia only occur in humans with rabies, but are neither sufficiently sensitive nor specific. The confusion between N-*methyl-D-aspartate receptor* (NMDAR) and limbic encephalitis and rabies is mechanistically coherent given the tropism of both diseases for limbic brain structures.[24] Rabies is commonly mistaken for cerebral malaria and may be coincident.[25] Rabies

Table 1
Exposures to rabies and rationale for investigation and postexposure prophylaxis

Exposure	Rationale	Action and Timing
Bite by a wild terrestrial mammal other than small rodent or lagomorph	Rabies is abundant in wildlife and cross-species transmission occurs.[75] Many small rodents and lagomorphs paralyze and die before salivary excretion of virus occurs.[76]	Sacrifice animal and submit head to public health authorities to test brain for rabies. Urgent PEP pending test results[a]
Unprovoked bite by a pet (dog, cat, or ferret)	Pet vaccination is imperfect.[20] Cross-species transmission occurs. Incubation periods are well-defined.	Observation for 10 d[b,c] Urgent PEP if animal has rabies
Unprovoked bite by a domestic mammal (horse, cow, or other pet)	Vaccinations exist for horses, cattle, and sheep, but efficacy and incubation period are poorly defined.	Report the incident to the local public health department. The animal may be sacrificed and the head submitted for testing.[b] Urgent PEP
Dog or cat brings live prey to their master.	Without direct bite by the prey, there is no human exposure. The dog or cat is exposed.	Sacrifice the prey and submit for testing. If positive for rabies, boost a vaccinated pet and quarantine for 45 d.[2] Sacrifice an unvaccinated pet.
Dog or cat brings dead, desiccated prey to their master.	Virus is rapidly inactivated by desiccation or sunlight– no exposure.	No action
Physical contact with a bat	Bat bites are hard to appreciate or find by examination. Most American deaths from bat rabies have no known exposure, so known exposure confers very high odds for death from rabies.	Sacrifice animal and submit for testing. If positive or if animal cannot be tested, urgent PEP
Bat seen in the same room as a responsible child (>6 y) or adult	Physical contact can be reliably excluded – no exposure	No action
Bat seen in the same room as a young child (<7 y),[d] sleeping, intoxicated or cognitively impaired person	Eight percent of bats found indoors are rabid.[77] Physical contact CANNOT be reliably excluded – exposure occurred	Sacrifice animal and submit for testing. If positive or if animal cannot be tested, urgent PEP
Bat found in a room that was previously occupied or seen in a hallway or room adjacent to persons who cannot report physical contact with a bat.	Risk of undetected contact is substantially lower – no exposure	No action

[a] It may be worth completing a pre-exposure prophylaxis series (0, 7, 21, or 28) if testing results negative because repeat exposures may be anticipated and if insurance/finances permit.
[b] Quarantine and sacrifice can only be imposed by public health authorities.
[c] Quarantine for 45 days and revaccinate pet if pet was vaccinated for rabies but immunization has lapsed.
[d] Untruths are common by young children seeking to please or avoid punishment. The age for informed assent was arbitrarily chosen as cutoff.

Box 2
Mimics of rabies

1. NMDAR-antibody mediated encephalitis and limbic encephalitis

2. Cerebral malaria

3. Conversion disorders, delirium, and acute psychotic disorders

4. Postvaccinal encephalitis

5. Herpes simplex encephalitis

6. Scorpion and elapid (snake) envenomations

7. Illicit drug use

8. Organophosphate poisoning

9. Tetanus

10. Guillain-Barré syndrome, brachial neuritis, and *Campylobacter*-associated summer paralysis syndrome

---

patients are often referred to psychiatric hospitals[26] and it is common for rabies-exposed individuals to develop focal neurologic symptoms after PEP.[27] Elapid (snake) toxins share amino acid homology with the attachment glycoprotein of rabies virus[28] whereas scorpion envenomations cause a clinical syndrome overlapping with rabies.[29] Transplantation-associated outbreaks of rabies have been associated with the diagnosis of illicit drug use or other intoxication of the donor.[30–32]

The absence of a history of fever and a prolonged prodrome of more than 2 weeks make rabies unlikely.[21] Cerebrospinal fluid (CSF) analyses and neuroimaging are subtly abnormal normal at time of presentation with rabies.[33] Grossly purulent CSF or MRIs involving mostly white matter lesions or contrast enhancement of any lesion are inconsistent with early rabies.

Laboratory confirmation of rabies virus infection is absolutely necessary because of the implications of the diagnosis to the patient and the patient's family, to physicians contemplating imminent treatment or palliation, and for protection of medical staff and contacts. Laboratory diagnosis requires detection of the virus or host response to the virus by a panel of tests, all imperfect but in aggregate detecting 90% of human rabies (**Box 3**).[21] Repeat testing is often needed to improve test sensitivity. Polymerase chain reaction (PCR) detection in skin and saliva is highly sensitive, but genetic variability of rabies virus and other lyssaviruses requires that multiple primer sets be considered. Corneal imprints are no longer recommended for diagnosis of rabies because of the risk of the procedure and poor accuracy. Immune response to rabies antigens can be detected at time of presentation in bat rabies but is rarely present in dog rabies before 5 days of hospitalization. The immune response to rabies is usually present by 14 days of hospitalization unless immunosuppressive disease or therapies (including ribavirin) were involved.[21,34,35] Diagnosis of rabies requires expert reference laboratories and may take several days to result. Technologies, such as NMR metabolomics, show promise for early, specific diagnosis of rabies in less specialized laboratories.[36]

PROGNOSIS

Modern PEP has never failed in the United States since the introduction of cell-based vaccines in the mid-1970s, assuming prompt but not necessarily emergent application of PEP.[37] Rabies PEP is costly and can be averted if the animal is submitted for testing

---

Box 3
Diagnosis of rabies

A. Exposure to an animal bite or rabies virus-infected saliva, AND

B. Clinical syndrome of acute, rapidly progressive encephalitis or acute flaccid paralysis syndrome, AND

C. Laboratory confirmation by rabies

     a. Biopsy of hairy skin (nape of neck)

        i. Detection of rabies RNA by PCR (60%–100% sensitivity[78,79])

        ii. Detection of rabies antigen by DFA (67% sensitivity[21])

     b. Saliva

        i. Detection of rabies RNA by PCR (58%–100% sensitivity when done serially[21,78–80])

        ii. Detection of infectious rabies virus by intracerebral inoculation into suckling mice (50% sensitivity)

        iii. Detection of rabies virus by tissue culture (60% sensitivity; 87% of seronegative patients[21])

     c. Blood

        i. Detection of total rabies antibodies by IFA (>90% sensitive after 14 days)

        ii. Detection of antirabies G glycoprotein antibodies by ELISA (>90% sensitive after 14 d[8,80])[a]

        iii. Detection of neutralizing antibodies to rabies by RFFIT, FAVN or similar assays (>90% sensitive after 14 d)

     d. CSF

        i. Detection of total rabies antibodies by IFA (>90% sensitive after 14 days)

        ii. Detection of antirabies G glycoprotein antibodies by ELISA (>90% sensitive after 14 days)[1]

        iii. Detection of neutralizing antibodies to rabies by RFFIT, FAVN, or similar assays (>90% sensitive after 14 days)

        iv. Detection of rabies RNA by PCR (very poor sensitivity)

     e. Biopsy of brain (antemortem)

        i. Detection of rabies RNA by PCR (75% sensitivity)

        ii. Detection of rabies antigen by DFA (100% sensitivity[21])

        iii. Detection of rabies virus by tissue culture (60% sensitivity)

     f. Corneal imprints – no longer recommended; risky

        i. Detection of rabies antigen in epithelial cells by DFA (28% sensitivity[21])

Abbreviations: DFA, direct fluorescent antibody; FAVN, fluorescent antibody virus neutralization; IFA, immunofluorescent antibody; RFFIT, rapid fluorescent focus inhibition test.

[a] Rabies antibody detection by ELISA is approved for demonstration of a proxy of immunity in human serum in many countries but is not an approved diagnostic test for human rabies. It has been used, off label, in some countries in serum and CSF for this purpose.

---

and tests negative for rabies. The rare failure of PEP usually involves highly traumatic bites about the face and neck that correspond to heavy innervation density, short axonal lengths, and short incubation periods.[38] Both rabies immune globulin (RIG) and rabies vaccine are necessary to prevent rabies.

Rabies remains statistically 100% fatal, with more than 50,000 patients diagnosed annually and fewer than 20 known survivors over the past 50 years.[39] Most of these are recent survivors. Some survivors may not be true rabies survivors but rather meet current definitions of human rabies (see **Box 3**), such as having antibodies against rabies nucleoprotein but without the neutralizing antibodies that should predict survival. In some instances, exhaustive investigations to determine alternative diagnoses to rabies were unfruitful.[19] Alternatively, as is true in many animal species, rabies virus may cause a continuum of severity of disease.[40] Among known rabies survivors associated with the Milwaukee protocol, there seems to be a dichotomy of outcomes, with 4 showing nearly full neurologic recovery and 4 having profound, permanent neurologic deficits or later demise.[41]

MANAGEMENT

The 4 keys to prophylaxis of a bite or lick from a rabies-infected mammal include (1) generous lavage of the bite wound with soap or topical antiseptic and water and (2) avoidance of definitive wound repair. Many of these wounds become bacterially infected when closed primarily, so haste in repair is short-sighted. It is better to use a few sutures to approximate wound edges, followed by more definitive and expert wound closure electively after 7 to 14 days. Tetanus prophylaxis is also indicated. (3) RIG is of human or modified-equine origin and is essential for bridging immunity until the response to rabies vaccination occurs at 10 to 14 days. RIG is most efficacious when infiltrated into the wound and does not usually produce detectable serum levels of antibody when given intramuscularly (IM), remote from the bite wound. The recommended dosage cannot be exceeded without interfering with vaccine take, but RIG can be diluted in saline to cover large wounds. RIG is not needed if the first rabies vaccine was administered more than 7 days before RIG administration because endogenous antibody production is then present, but the patient remains at risk of disease progression during this period, with rabies developing in the third or fourth week of PEP.

(4) Rabies vaccine should be a modern cell-based, inactivated vaccine. Older nerve tissue–derived vaccines produce autoimmune neurologic syndromes with high attack rates (1:400–1:5000 persons) and confer only partial protection against rabies. It is advisable to seek pre-exposure prophylaxis before trips to (or living in) rabies endemic areas where access to rabies vaccine and RIG, in particular, is limited, and to change travel plans to seek modern PEP if attacked by a potentially rabid animal. Although RIG and immunization provide the most benefit when given within days of rabies exposure, the incubation period for rabies can be long and travelers may still benefit from delayed immunization at any time after an encounter, even past 1 year.

Rabies vaccine is effective when given intradermally (ID) or IM, although only the latter route is licensed in the United States. ID routes are cost effective when used in specialized dog-bite clinics in endemic areas. There are several schemata for immunization recommended by the World Health Organization (WHO). In the United States, only 4 doses (from the original 6) are now recommended (0, 3, 7, and 14 days) because an immune response is invariably present by day 14.[42] The immunologic rationale for the day 3 dose is unclear and not used in the Zagreb (WHO) 0, 7, and 21 days IM scheme or the 4-site and 8-site (non-WHO) 0, 7, and 28 days ID schemata.[43] Extra doses of rabies vaccine have been hard to eliminate when prophylaxis is indicated for a highly fatal condition.

Although many antivirals are effective in vitro against the rabies virus, there are no known effective antivirals for treating the disease. There is no benefit to use of RIG or inactivated rabies vaccine when treating symptomatic patients. In the Milwaukee protocol, use of ribavirin, amantadine, and ketamine did not alter salivary viral loads. (Ribavirin is no longer used in the protocol.) Use of interferon alpha and interferon inducers (inosiplex and poly I-C) have not been effective and even seem to potentiate brain damage.[44–46] Interferon beta is licensed for CNS diseases but has not been studied to treat rabies. Brain cooling has been proposed to treat rabies but has not been successful in several instances.[47]

COMPLICATIONS

Rabies usually results in death. With increased attention to survival from rabies, natural survivors have recently been reported from India, with poor functional outcomes.[48,49] Four survivors using the Milwaukee protocol have had excellent cognitive outcomes, although 2 had spastic diplegia (similar to what has been described in survivors of animal models of rabies).[40]

Critical care prolongs survival and has permitted further characterization of the later clinical course of rabies; 20% of patients die after cardiac arrest or other dysrhythmia within the first week of symptom onset, which can be avoided by sedation.[50] Most rabies patients have modest initial increases in intracranial pressure that are not visible by CT or MRI and correlate with increased concentrations of N-acetylaspartate (NAA) in CSF.[36] Six to 8 days after hospitalization, patients develop dysautonomia and coma. This event has correlated in some patients with moderate to severe spasm of the intracranial arteries measured by transcranial Doppler (TCD) ultrasound and with metabolic changes in the CSF measured by nuclear magnetic resonance (NMR).[51,52] The cerebral dysautonomia resolves spontaneously and no lesions are evident at later autopsy. A second period of dysautonomia follows 12 to 15 days after hospitalization and is frequently catastrophic. Intracranial blood velocities by TCD and intracranial pressure by invasive monitoring drop acutely, indicating loss of cerebral blood volume. The electroencephalogram loses activity, pupils dilate, and diabetes insipidus follows within 24 hours. Cerebral edema develops in some patients after the event. Patients then die unresponsive to aggressive medical interventions. Again, there is no vascular lesion at autopsy.

Some patients recover from rabies with supportive critical care and an early and vigorous immune response to the rabies virus. Survivors rapidly regain neurologic function.[53] The immune response to rabies has been associated with complications, such as complete heart block in 40% of patients with dog rabies and prolonged cerebral edema in patients with bat rabies. The mechanisms behind these rabies virus phylogeny-specific complications and whether they are part of an immune response to the rabies virus are unclear.

EVIDENCE

The true burden of rabies in the world is unknown. Rabies is a disease of poor, marginalized, and geographically isolated populations. The burden of rabies is extrapolated from rates of dog bites treated at hospitals and specialized clinics and by estimated rates of rabies among dogs in these areas.[39] The underestimation of rabies burden may be considerable if the continuum of disease severity caused by rabies virus is wide[11–13] and includes asymptomatic disease in indigenous populations.[15,17]

The evidence behind PEP is strong but antedates controlled clinical trials. Equivalency studies using immunologic endpoints justify different PEP regimens.[43] There is no immunologic correlate of rabies protection.

The evidence for treatment of rabies is extremely poor, although with more attempts at treating rabies and more prolonged survival, the opportunity to put rabies therapeutics on sound scientific footage has never been greater. There is probably ethical equipoise in comparing conventional critical care to the Milwaukee protocol for treatment of rabies.

CONTROVERSIES

The basic science of rabies is muddied by more than a century of reliance on fixed rabies virus strains that were laboratory -adapted to the point of displaying biological properties (cell specificity, incubation period, cytopathic effect, and immunogenicity) that are almost diametrically opposite to those of wild-type strains. Although these mutants are useful for theoretic virology and for scalable production of inactivated vaccine strains, they are regularly misleading about rabies pathogenesis. Studies of wild-type rabies viruses of different phylogenies in survival animal models are desperately needed to further rabies therapeutics and clarify the field.

It is embarrassing that rabies has been vaccine-preventable since the 1800s, yet rabies is emergent today. Rabies remains a disease of poverty and is even neglected among neglected tropical diseases. There are 2 economic challenges to preventing rabies. The first is that rabies is a zoonosis, which therefore spans a wide governmental chasm. Interventions to prevent or treat rabies by public health ministries are cost ineffective relative to vector control, whereas control of rabies vectors through vaccination and fertility control have trouble being justified solely by agricultural or wildlife burden within ministries of agriculture and environment.[54] The second economic and ethical challenge is that the cost of prophylaxis is high and out of range for most populations. There is considerable irony that pre-exposure prophylaxis is recommended for child travelers to or child expatriates living in rabies endemic areas where routine childhood vaccination against rabies is not practiced. Feasibility studies of rabies vaccination as a component of a childhood vaccination schedule recur regularly,[55–59] and the use of rabies vaccine as a control for field-testing malaria vaccines is encouraging.[60] There is some hope that the cost of rabies biologicals will fall soon given regional development of attenuated and inactivated live vaccines, ID routes of vaccine administration, recombinant vectors, DNA vaccines, and monoclonal antibodies.[43,61–72]

The Milwaukee protocol relies on critical care and metabolic support to treat rabies in the absence of effective antivirals. Seven additional survivors are known after 48 known attempts (14.6% survival) by intention to treat.[41] The protocol remains highly controversial because the approach is aggressive and the mechanism of benefit is unclear.[47,73] The concept of a possible continuum of rabies disease severity supports further attempts at nonspecific critical care of rabies, because critical care is well suited to shifting a continuum of severity toward increased survival. Whether specific components of the Milwaukee protocol provide benefit over conventional critical care will require randomized trials.

Rabies seems as much an acquired metabolic disorder as a conventional viral disease, because rabies is poorly cytopathic and poorly inflammatory. The delay of several days between massive CNS infection by rabies virus and onset of clinical symptoms and signs is consistent with an acquired metabolic disorder involving accumulation (increased concentration of NAA) or depletion (deficiency of tetrahydrobiopterin [BH$_4$]) of metabolites. The rapid neurologic recovery after rabies and the lack of histologic damage at autopsy (cytopathic effect by rabies virus or the immune response) at autopsy also support a metabolic mechanism of neurologic dysfunction. NMR studies of CSF during treatment of rabies define a metabolomics profile of rabies encephalitis and also document a reversal in metabolic derangements among rabies survivors.[36] A severe deficiency of BH_4 has also been described in human rabies.[74] BH_4 is an enzyme cofactor essential for the synthesis of neurotransmitters, including dopamine, norepinephrine, serotonin, and nitric oxide. Recovery after rabies is accelerated by supplementation with BH_4 (sapropterin).

REFERENCES

1. Smith JS, Fishbein DB, Rupprecht CE, et al. Unexplained rabies in three immigrants in the United States. A virologic investigation. N Engl J Med 1991;324: 205–11.
2. Hemachudha T, Ugolini G, Wacharapluesadee S, et al. Human rabies: neuropathogenesis, diagnosis, and management. Lancet Neurol 2013;12:498–513.
3. Centers for Disease Control and Prevention (CDC). Human rabies - Kentucky/Indiana, 2009. MMWR Morb Mortal Wkly Rep 2010;59:393–6.
4. Laothamatas J, Wacharapluesadee S, Lumlertdacha B, et al. Furious and paralytic rabies of canine origin: neuroimaging with virological and cytokine studies. J Neurovirol 2008;14:119–29.
5. Hemachudha T, Sunsaneewitayakul B, Mitrabhakdi E, et al. Paralytic complications following intravenous rabies immune globulin treatment in a patient with furious rabies. Int J Infect Dis 2003;7:76–7.
6. Lodmell DL, Bell JF, Moore GJ, et al. Comparative study of abortive and nonabortive rabies in mice. J Infect Dis 1969;119:569–80.
7. Galelli A, Baloul L, Lafon M. Abortive rabies virus central nervous infection is controlled by T lymphocyte local recruitment and induction of apoptosis. J Neurovirol 2000;6:359–72.
8. Caicedo Y, Paez A, Kuzmin I, et al. Virology, immunology and pathology of human rabies during treatment. Pediatr Infect Dis J 2015;34:520–8.
9. Hunter M, Johnson N, Hedderwick S, et al. Immunovirological correlates in human rabies treated with therapeutic coma. J Med Virol 2010;82:1255–65.
10. Hooper DC, Morimoto K, Bette M, et al. Collaboration of antibody and inflammation in clearance of rabies virus from the central nervous system. J Virol 1998;72:3711–9.
11. Holzmann-Pazgal G, Wanger A, Degaffe G, et al. Presumptive abortive human rabies - Texas, 2009. MMWR Morb Mortal Wkly Rep 2010;59:185–90.
12. Rawat AK, Rao SK. Survival of a rabies patient. Indian Pediatr 2011;48:574.
13. Karahocagil MK, Akdeniz H, Aylan O, et al. Complete recovery from clinical rabies: case report. Turkiye Klinikleri Journal of Medical Science 2013;33:547–52.
14. Phares TW, Kean RB, Mikheeva T, et al. Regional differences in blood-brain barrier permeability changes and inflammation in the apathogenic clearance of virus from the central nervous system. J Immunol 2006;176:7666–75.
15. Gilbert AT, Petersen BW, Recuenco S, et al. Evidence of rabies virus exposure among humans in the Peruvian Amazon. Am J Trop Med Hyg 2012;87:206–15.
16. Follmann EH, Ritter DG, Beller M. Survey of fox trappers in northern Alaska for rabies antibody. Epidemiol Infect 1994;113:137–41.
17. Orr PH, Rubin MR, Aoki FY. Naturally acquired serum rabies neutralizing antibody in a Canadian Inuit population. Arctic Med Res 1988;47(Suppl 1):699–700.
18. Black D, Wiktor TJ. Survey of raccoon hunters for rabies antibody titers: pilot study. J Fla Med Assoc 1986;73:517–20.
19. Wiedeman J, Plant J, Glaser C, et al. Recovery of a patient from clinical rabies–California, 2011. MMWR Morb Mortal Wkly Rep 2012;61:61–5.
20. Murray KO, Holmes KC, Hanlon CA. Rabies in vaccinated dogs and cats in the United States, 1997-2001. J Am Vet Med Assoc 2009;235:691–5.

21. Noah DL, Drenzek CL, Smith JS, et al. Epidemiology of human rabies in the United States, 1980 to 1996. Ann Intern Med 1998;128:922–30.
22. Manning SE, Rupprecht CE, Fishbein D, et al. Human rabies prevention–United States, 2008: recommendations of the Advisory Committee on Immunization Practices. MMWR Recomm Rep 2008;57:1–28.
23. De Serres G, Skowronski DM, Mimault P, et al. Bats in the Bedroom, Bats in the Belfry: reanalysis of the Rationale for Rabies Postexposure Prophylaxis. Clin Infect Dis 2009;48:1493–9.
24. Gable MS, Gavali S, Radner A, et al. Anti-NMDA receptor encephalitis: report of ten cases and comparison with viral encephalitis. Eur J Clin Microbiol Infect Dis 2009;28:1421–9.
25. Mallewa M, Vallely P, Faragher B, et al. Viral CNS infections in children from a malaria-endemic area of Malawi: a prospective cohort study. Lancet Glob Health 2013;1:e153–60.
26. Punja M, Pomerleau AC, Devlin JJ, et al. Anti-N-methyl-D-aspartate receptor (anti-NMDAR) encephalitis: an etiology worth considering in the differential diagnosis of delirium. Clin Toxicol (Phila) 2013;51:794–7.
27. Mattner F, Bitz F, Goedecke M, et al. Adverse effects of rabies pre- and postexposure prophylaxis in 290 health-care-workers exposed to a rabies infected organ donor or transplant recipients. Infection 2007;35:219–24.
28. Lentz TL, Wilson PT, Hawrot E, et al. Amino acid sequence similarity between rabies virus glycoprotein and snake venom curaremimetic neurotoxins. Science 1984;226:847–8.
29. Boyer LV, Theodorou AA, Berg RA, et al. Antivenom for critically ill children with neurotoxicity from scorpion stings. N Engl J Med 2009;360:2090–8.
30. Srinivasan A, Burton EC, Kuehnert MJ, et al. Transmission of rabies virus from an organ donor to four transplant recipients. N Engl J Med 2005;352:1103–11.
31. Maier T, Schwarting A, Mauer D, et al. Management and outcomes after multiple corneal and solid organ transplantations from a donor infected with rabies virus. Clin Infect Dis 2010;50:1112–9.
32. Vora NM, Basavaraju SV, Feldman KA, et al. Raccoon rabies virus variant transmission through solid organ transplantation. JAMA 2013;310:398–407.
33. Laothamatas J, Hemachudha T, Mitrabhakdi E, et al. MR imaging in human rabies. AJNR Am J Neuroradiol 2003;24:1102–9.
34. Anderson LJ, Nicholson KG, Tauxe RV, et al. Human rabies in the United States, 1960 to 1979: epidemiology, diagnosis, and prevention. Ann Intern Med 1984; 100:728–35.
35. Powers CN, Peavy DL, Knight V. Selective inhibition of functional lymphocyte subpopulations by ribavirin. Antimicrob Agents Chemother 1982;22:108–14.
36. O'Sullivan A, Willoughby RE, Mishchuk D, et al. Metabolomics of cerebrospinal fluid from humans treated for rabies. J Proteome Res 2013;12:481–90.
37. Rupprecht CE, Gibbons RV. Clinical practice. Prophylaxis against rabies. N Engl J Med 2004;351:2626–35.
38. Hemachudha T, Mitrabhakdi E, Wilde H, et al. Additional reports of failure to respond to treatment after rabies exposure in Thailand. Clin Infect Dis 1999;28: 143–4.
39. Knobel DL, Cleaveland S, Coleman PG, et al. Re-evaluating the burden of rabies in Africa and Asia. Bull World Health Organ 2005;83:360–8.
40. Feder HM Jr, Petersen BW, Robertson KL, et al. Rabies: still a uniformly fatal disease? Historical occurrence, epidemiological trends, and paradigm shifts. Curr Infect Dis Rep 2012;14:408–22.

41. Willoughby RE Jr. Rabies treatment protocol and registry. Milwaukee (WI): Medical College of Wisconsin and Children's Hospital of Wisconsin; 2013. Available at: www.mcw.edu/rabies.
42. Rupprecht CE, Briggs D, Brown CM, et al. Use of a reduced (4-dose) vaccine schedule for postexposure prophylaxis to prevent human rabies: recommendations of the advisory committee on immunization practices. MMWR Recomm Rep 2010;59:1–9.
43. Warrell MJ. Current rabies vaccines and prophylaxis schedules: preventing rabies before and after exposure. Travel Med Infect Dis 2012;10:1–15.
44. Warrell MJ, White NJ, Looareesuwan S, et al. Failure of interferon alfa and tribavirin in rabies encephalitis. BMJ 1989;299:830–3.
45. Dolman CL, Charlton KM. Massive necrosis of the brain in rabies. Can J Neurol Sci 1987;14:162–5.
46. Gode GR, Saksena R, Batra RK, et al. Treatment of 54 clinically diagnosed rabies patients with two survivals. Indian J Med Res 1988;88:564–6.
47. Jackson AC. Current and future approaches to the therapy of human rabies. Antiviral Res 2013;99:61–7.
48. de Souza A, Madhusudana SN. Survival from rabies encephalitis. J Neurol Sci 2014;339:8–14.
49. Karande S, Muranjan M, Mani RS, et al. Atypical rabies encephalitis in a six-year-old boy: clinical, radiological, and laboratory findings. Int J Infect Dis 2015;36:1–3.
50. Schankin CJ, Birnbaum T, Linn J, et al. A fatal encephalitis. Lancet 2005;365:358.
51. Coen M, O'Sullivan M, Bubb WA, et al. Proton nuclear magnetic resonance-based metabonomics for rapid diagnosis of meningitis and ventriculitis. Clin Infect Dis 2005;41:1582–90.
52. Willoughby RE, Roy-Burman A, Martin KW, et al. Generalized cranial artery spasm in human rabies. Dev Biol (Basel) 2008;131:367–75.
53. Willoughby RE Jr, Tieves KS, Hoffman GM, et al. Survival after treatment of rabies with induction of coma. N Engl J Med 2005;352:2508–14.
54. Reece JF, Chawla SK, Hiby AR. Decline in human dog-bite cases during a street dog sterilisation programme in Jaipur, India. Vet Rec 2013;172:473.
55. Fooks AR, Koraka P, de Swart RL, et al. Development of a multivalent paediatric human vaccine for rabies virus in combination with Measles-Mumps-Rubella (MMR). Vaccine 2014;32:2020–1.
56. Malerczyk C, Vakil HB, Bender W. Rabies pre-exposure vaccination of children with purified chick embryo cell vaccine (PCECV). Hum Vaccin Immunother 2013;9:1454–9.
57. Shanbag P, Shah N, Kulkarni M, et al. Protecting Indian Schoolchildren against rabies: pre-exposure vaccination with purified chick embryo cell vaccine (PCECV) or purified verocell rabies vaccine (PVRV). Hum Vaccin 2008;4:365–9.
58. Sabchareon A, Chantavanich P, Pasuralertsakul S, et al. Persistence of antibodies in children after intradermal or intramuscular administration of preexposure primary and booster immunizations with purified Vero cell rabies vaccine. Pediatr Infect Dis J 1998;17:1001–7.
59. Lang J, Duong GH, Nguyen VG, et al. Randomised feasibility trial of pre-exposure rabies vaccination with DTP-IPV in infants. Lancet 1997;349:1663–5.
60. Bejon P, Lusingu J, Olotu A, et al. Efficacy of RTS,S/AS01E vaccine against malaria in children 5 to 17 months of age. N Engl J Med 2008;359:2521–32.

61. Nagarajan T, Rupprecht CE, Dessain SK, et al. Human monoclonal antibody and vaccine approaches to prevent human rabies. Curr Top Microbiol Immunol 2008; 317:67–101.
62. Ravish HS, Srikanth J, Ashwath Narayana DH, et al. Pre-exposure prophylaxis against rabies in children: safety of purified chick embryo cell rabies vaccine (Vaxirab N) when administered by intradermal route. Hum Vaccin Immunother 2013;9:1910–3.
63. Saxena S, Sonwane AA, Dahiya SS, et al. Induction of immune responses and protection in mice against rabies using a self-replicating RNA vaccine encoding rabies virus glycoprotein. Vet Microbiol 2009;136:36–44.
64. Li R, Huang L, Li J, et al. A next-generation, serum-free, highly purified Vero cell rabies vaccine is safe and as immunogenic as the reference vaccine Verorab(R) when administered according to a post-exposure regimen in healthy children and adults in China. Vaccine 2013;31:5940–7.
65. Zhou M, Zhang G, Ren G, et al. Recombinant rabies viruses expressing GM-CSF or flagellin are effective vaccines for both intramuscular and oral immunizations. PLoS One 2013;8:e63384.
66. Zhang S, Liu Y, Fooks AR, et al. Oral vaccination of dogs (Canis familiaris) with baits containing the recombinant rabies-canine adenovirus type-2 vaccine confers long-lasting immunity against rabies. Vaccine 2008;26:345–50.
67. Koraka P, Bosch BJ, Cox M, et al. A recombinant rabies vaccine expressing the trimeric form of the glycoprotein confers enhanced immunogenicity and protection in outbred mice. Vaccine 2014;32:4644–50.
68. Both L, van DC, Wright E, et al. Production, characterization, and antigen specificity of recombinant 62-71-3, a candidate monoclonal antibody for rabies prophylaxis in humans. FASEB J 2013;27:2055–65.
69. Gogtay N, Thatte U, Kshirsagar N, et al. Safety and pharmacokinetics of a human monoclonal antibody to rabies virus: a randomized, dose-escalation phase 1 study in adults. Vaccine 2012;30:7315–20.
70. Kaku Y, Noguchi A, Hotta K, et al. Inhibition of rabies virus propagation in mouse neuroblastoma cells by an intrabody against the viral phosphoprotein. Antiviral Res 2011;91:64–71.
71. Bakker AB, Python C, Kissling CJ, et al. First administration to humans of a monoclonal antibody cocktail against rabies virus: safety, tolerability, and neutralizing activity. Vaccine 2008;26:5922–7.
72. Sloan SE, Hanlon C, Weldon W, et al. Identification and characterization of a human monoclonal antibody that potently neutralizes a broad panel of rabies virus isolates. Vaccine 2007;25:2800–10.
73. Wilde H, Wacharapluesadee S, Saraya A, et al. Human rabies prevention (comment from a canine-rabies-endemic region). J Travel Med 2013;20: 139–42.
74. Willoughby RE Jr, Opladen T, Maier T, et al. Tetrahydrobiopterin deficiency in human rabies. J Inherit Metab Dis 2008;32:65–72.
75. Wallace RM, Gilbert A, Slate D, et al. Right place, wrong species: a 20-year review of rabies virus cross species transmission among terrestrial mammals in the United States. PLoS One 2014;9:e107539.
76. Eidson M, Matthews SD, Willsey AL, et al. Rabies virus infection in a pet guinea pig and seven pet rabbits. J Am Vet Med Assoc 2005;227:932–5, 918.
77. Robbins A, Eidson M, Keegan M, et al. Bat incidents at children's camps, New York State, 1998-2002. Emerg Infect Dis 2005;11:302–5.

78. Mani RS, Madhusudana SN, Mahadevan A, et al. Utility of real-time Taqman PCR for antemortem and postmortem diagnosis of human rabies. J Med Virol 2014;86: 1804–12.
79. Dacheux L, Reynes JM, Buchy P, et al. A reliable diagnosis of human rabies based on analysis of skin biopsy specimens. Clin Infect Dis 2008;47:1410–7.
80. Hemachudha T, Wacharapluesadee S. Antemortem diagnosis of human rabies. Clin Infect Dis 2004;39:1085–6.

The Challenge of Global Poliomyelitis Eradication

Julie R. Garon, MPH[a], Stephen L. Cochi, MD, MPH[b],
Walter A. Orenstein, MD[a],*

KEYWORDS

- Poliomyelitis • Eradication • Oral poliovirus vaccine (OPV)
- Inactivated poliovirus vaccine (IPV)

KEY POINTS

- More than 99% of poliomyelitis cases are asymptomatic or consist of mild illness without paralysis. Acute Flaccid Paralysis (AFP), a sign of polio, is also a sign of many other diseases.
- Physicians should suspect polio in a clinically compatible case. There may not be a history of travel to a polio endemic/epidemic country as the person transmitting virus to the paralytic case could have had an asymptomatic infection or nonparalytic illness.
- A single case of paralytic polio demands immediate attention, including notification of the state health department and Centers for Disease Control and Prevention (CDC) and collection of stool samples for laboratory confirmation.
- Since 1988, the number of poliomyelitis cases has been reduced by more than 99%, yet reservoirs of disease remain. Barriers to eradication include insecurity, political commitment, and immunization system quality.
- US physicians play an important role in surveillance, vaccination, advocacy, and financial support for global eradication of polio.

Disclosure Statement: W.A. Orenstein and J.R. Garon are supported by the Bill & Melinda Gates Foundation under Work Order 23848 awarded to the Task Force for Global Health. Apart from those disclosed, the authors do not have any conflicts of interest to report and do not have relevant affiliations, relationships, or financial involvement with organizations with a financial interest in materials disclosed in the article. No writing assistance was used in the production of this article.

[a] Division of Infectious Diseases, Emory University School of Medicine, 1462 Clifton Road Northeast, Suite 446, Atlanta, GA 30322, USA; [b] Global Immunization Division, Center for Global Health Centers for Disease Control and Prevention, 1600 Clifton Road Northeast, Mailstop A-04, Atlanta, GA 30333, USA
* Corresponding author.
E-mail address: worenst@emory.edu

Infect Dis Clin N Am 29 (2015) 651–665
http://dx.doi.org/10.1016/j.idc.2015.07.003
0891-5520/15/$ – see front matter © 2015 Elsevier Inc. All rights reserved.

INTRODUCTION

Today, few Americans may remember the devastating implications and fear caused by poliomyelitis outbreaks given that there has not been an outbreak of paralytic polio in the United States since 1979. Before the development of effective vaccines, poliomyelitis was a seasonal epidemic disease in the United States. The number of cases peaked in 1952 when more than 20,000 cases of paralytic polio were reported.[1] Although some people recovered from paralytic polio, many suffered permanent paralysis and even death. Hospital wards filled with iron lungs and permanently disabled children served as painful visible reminders to society of the toll this debilitating disease took on young lives. With an estimated 350,000 polio cases worldwide and endemic disease in 125 countries the World Health Assembly launched the Global Polio Eradication Initiative (GPEI) in 1988, targeting the disease for eradication.

POLIO AS A CANDIDATE FOR ERADICATION

Global eradication is currently defined as, "the worldwide absence of a specific disease agent in nature as a result of deliberate control efforts that may be discontinued where the agent is judged no longer to present a significant risk from extrinsic sources."[2] Determining if a disease is a good candidate for eradication depends on whether or not it meets 4 key criteria. These criteria include the following:

1. Humans are required to maintain the pathogen.
2. Sensitive and specific diagnostic tools are available.
3. There is an effective intervention to terminate human-to-human transmission.
4. There is proof of principle (ie, elimination of transmission in a large geographic area).

Poliovirus requires a specific cell receptor (PVR or CD155) for infection that is expressed only on human and simian cells.[3] Therefore, humans are the only host for sustained poliovirus transmission as primate population sizes are too small to maintain sustained transmission. Breaking the chains of human-to-human transmission can eradicate the virus. Although asymptomatic cases present a challenge to surveillance, AFP reporting and virologic testing of stool are reliable ways to detect polio cases in populations. Although not without certain limitations, oral poliovirus vaccine (OPV) and inactivated poliovirus vaccine (IPV) are effective tools in preventing infection in individuals and reducing circulation of poliovirus within communities. With its low cost, ease of administration, and ability to induce mucosal immunity, OPV has been a particularly useful tool in interruption of transmission in populations. Lastly, early elimination of polio in the Western hemisphere served as proof of principle that eradication was possible throughout the world.

CLINICAL ASPECTS OF POLIO

Polioviruses, consisting of 3 antigenic types (serotypes 1, 2, and 3), are positive-sense single-stranded RNA Enteroviruses belonging to the Picornaviridae family.[3] Most poliovirus infections occur after oral ingestion of the virus followed by replication in the oral and intestinal mucosa, and most infections are asymptomatic.[3] In less than 1% of infections, the virus attacks the motor neurons of the anterior horn cells in the spinal cord, leading to destruction of those cells resulting in permanent paralysis of muscles. The most common cause of death from polio is respiratory insufficiency, when the infection affects respiratory muscles, occurring in about 5% to 10% of cases.[3,4] There is absence of sensory abnormalities, although deep tendon reflexes may be absent as a result of the impact of infection on muscle function. Nerve conduction and electromyographic studies have determined destruction of the anterior horn cells of the spinal cord to be the anatomic location of paralysis.[5] The potential clinical course of poliovirus infections is summarized in **Table 1**.[3]

Paralytic polio is estimated to occur in 1 in 100 to 1 in 2000 infections (average, 1 in 200). Type 1 is the most neurovirulent virus, whereas type 2 is least neurovirulent. AFP is not specific for polio, and there are many other causes of AFP.[6] Features of the 4 most common diagnoses to consider in the differential diagnosis of AFP can be seen in **Table 2**.

EPIDEMIOLOGY OF POLIO

Wild poliovirus (WPV) is transmitted through person-to-person contact through the fecal-oral or oral-oral routes.[3] Fecal-oral spread is most common in developing countries, whereas oral-oral transmission is probably the major mode of transmission in industrialized countries, with high standards of hygiene.[4] The incubation period is 3 to 6 days between infection and first symptoms (minor illness) and from 7 to 21 days from infection to onset of paralytic disease.[3] Individuals are most infectious immediately before and 1 to 2 weeks after the onset of paralytic disease.[3] Poliovirus is excreted for approximately 2 weeks in saliva and longer (3–6 weeks) in stool.[3] In immunodeficient persons, prolonged shedding (more than 6 months) or chronic excretion (more than 5 years) rarely can occur, although only 45 prolonged excretors have been identified to date, largely confined to high- and middle-upper-income countries.[3] Poliovirus transmission typically peaks in the warm, summer months in temperate climates, which is why eradication efforts attempt to boost population immunity through vaccination campaigns during the cooler low season to interrupt transmission.

Molecular methods such as genomic sequencing have further contributed to the understanding of poliovirus transmission and epidemiology. As the WPV genotype naturally evolves at a rate of around 1% nucleotide substitutions per site per year, lineages can be tracked to further map geographic transmission and identify gaps in

Table 1
Clinical description of poliomyelitis

Consequence	Symptoms	Infections (%)
Inapparent infection without symptoms	None	72
Minor illness	Transient illness; 1–3 d fever, malaise, drowsiness, headache, nausea, vomiting, constipation, or sore throat, in various combinations	24
Nonparalytic poliomyelitis (aseptic meningitis)	Minor illness characterized as fever, sore throat, vomiting, malaise; 1–2 d later stiffness of neck or back; vomiting, severe headache, pain in limbs, back neck (lasts 2–10 d, recovery is usually rapid and complete)	4
Paralytic poliomyelitis	Minor illness for several days, symptom-free period of 1–3 d, followed by rapid onset of flaccid paralysis with fever and progression to maximum extent of paralysis within a few days	<1

Data from Sutter RW, Kew OM, Cochi SL, et al. 28 - Poliovirus vaccine—live. In: Plotkin SA, Orenstein WA, Offit PA, editors. Vaccines (sixth edition). London: W.B. Saunders; 2013. p. 598–645.

Table 2
Distinguishing features of 4 common diagnoses of AFP

	Poliomyelitis	Guillain-Barré Syndrome	Traumatic Neuritis (After Injection)	Transverse Myelitis
Paralysis	Development of paralysis 24- to 48-h onset to full paralysis; descending; reduced or absent muscle tone in affected limbs; decreased or absent deep tendon reflexes; cranial nerve involvement and respiratory insufficiency only when bulbar involvement present	Development of paralysis from hours to 10 d; ascending; global hypotonia; globally absent deep tendon reflexes; cramps; tingling; hypoesthesia of palms and soles; cranial nerve involvement often present, affecting nerves VII, IX, X, XI, XII	Development of paralysis from hours to 4 d; reduced or absent muscle tone in affected limb; decreased or absent deep tendon reflexes; hypothermia in affected limb	Development of paralysis from hours to 4 d; hypotonia in affected limbs; deep tendon reflexes absent in lower limbs early; hyperreflexia late; anesthesia of lower limbs with sensory level
Clinical features	High fever at onset; always present at onset of flaccid paralysis; gone when progression of paralysis stops; severe myalgia; backache	Respiratory insufficiency in severe cases, enhanced by bacterial pneumonia; frequent blood pressure alterations; sweating; blushing; body temperature fluctuations; transient bladder dysfunction	Fever common before, during, and after flaccid paralysis; pain in gluteus	Occasional respiratory insufficiency; autonomic signs and symptoms present; bladder dysfunction
Diagnostic tests	Inflammatory cerebrospinal fluid; abnormal nerve conduction velocity, third week: anterior horn cell disease (normal during first 2 wk); abnormal electromyography at 3 wk	Albumin-cytologic dissociation of cerebrospinal fluid; abnormal nerve conduction velocity; third week: slowed conduction; decreased motor amplitudes	Abnormal nerve conduction velocity, third week: axonal damage	Mild elevation in cells of cerebrospinal fluid
Sequelae at 3 mo and up to 1 y	Severe, asymmetric atrophy; skeletal deformities developing later	Symmetric atrophy of distal muscles	Moderate atrophy; only in affected limbs	Flaccid diplegia; atrophy after years

Adapted from Sutter RW, Kew OM, Cochi SL, et al. 28-Poliovirus vaccine—live, Table 28-3: distinguishing features of four common diagnoses of acute flaccid paralysis. In: Plotkin SA, Orenstein WA, Offit PA, editors. Vaccines (sixth edition). London: W.B. Saunders; 2013. p. 604; with permission.

surveillance.[3,7] Orphan viruses, denoted by more than 1.5% difference in nucleotide sequence in the VP1 region compared with other known viruses, can identify areas where viruses have been transmitting over time without being detected.[3]

PROGRESS TOWARD GLOBAL ERADICATION OF POLIO

In the last several years, WPV case counts have been at record lows, and Africa seems to be polio-free for the first time in history—as of July 28, 2015, the last case detected in Africa was in Somalia in August 2014.[8] Although hundreds of thousands of WPV cases were found globally 30 years ago, only 359 WPV cases were seen in 9 countries in 2014, and 34 cases as of July 28, 2015.[8] In 1988, 125 countries were considered endemic (never having interrupted poliovirus transmission), although only 3 are classified as such today (**Fig. 1**). All of the recent WPV cases reported are type 1. The last case of type 3 WPV was seen in November 2012, whereas the last naturally occurring case of type 2 WPV was found in 1999.[8] Of 6 World Health Organization (WHO) regions, 4 encompassing greater than 80% of the world's population have been certified polio free, meaning at least 3 years have passed in the presence of high-quality surveillance with no WPV cases occurring.

Although 2012 saw near cessation of international spread of WPV, 2013 brought an increase in cases with evidence that adult travelers were contributing. During the low season of 2014, WPV exportation occurred in several countries, leading the International Health Regulations Emergency Committee to declare the situation a "Public Health Emergency of International Concern" in May 2014[9]; this led to additional travel recommendations and increased vigilance among the global community.[10]

ERADICATION STRATEGIES

The main strategies for eradication up until this point have been ongoing strengthening of routine immunization coverage, continued supplementary immunization activities (SIAs), extensive surveillance to find the virus, and mopping up efforts in areas with

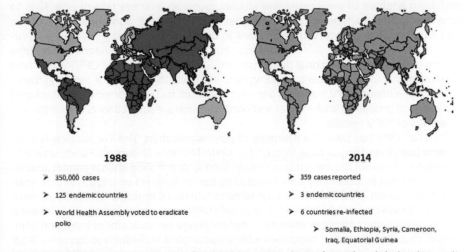

1988

> 350,000 cases

> 125 endemic countries

> World Health Assembly voted to eradicate polio

2014

> 359 cases reported

> 3 endemic countries

> 6 countries re-infected

> Somalia, Ethiopia, Syria, Cameroon, Iraq, Equatorial Guinea

Fig. 1. Progress in polio eradication from 1988 to 2014. (*Data from* The global polio eradication initiative. Data and Monitoring. 2015. Available at: http://www.polioeradication.org/ Dataandmonitoring.aspx. Accessed March 27, 2015.)

continued transmission. SIAs are mass vaccination campaigns conducted within a few days, multiple times a year, vaccinating all children less than 5 years regardless of vaccination history. Strategies such as finger and house marking can allow independent monitors to survey the area after the campaign to identify missed children and assess the quality of the campaign. Satellite and geographic information system technology have also been used to track vaccinators and further improve campaign quality.

AFP surveillance is the gold standard for detecting cases of polio. The Global Polio Laboratory Network consists of 146 WHO-accredited laboratories following standardized protocols for the following analyses: poliovirus detection by polymerase chain reaction and/or viral isolation, serotype, determination if the virus is wild or vaccine type (ie, wild or Sabin-like or vaccine-derived poliovirus [VDPV]), and genomic sequencing.[11] Sequencing results are closely analyzed by comparing nucleotide sequences in the VP1 coding region of isolates to track pathways of poliovirus transmission and guide vaccine choices and strategies through the last stages of the eradication program.[11] In addition to AFP surveillance, environmental surveillance is being increasingly used to monitor for the presence of poliovirus in pooled sewage or other environmental samples and to provide insight into international spread of the virus, particularly in areas in which termination of transmission has been difficult.

AVAILABLE VACCINES
Oral Poliovirus Vaccine

OPV consists of live attenuated polioviruses, originally developed by Albert Sabin. Multiple presentations of OPV are available, including trivalent OPV (tOPV) containing types 1, 2, and 3; bivalent OPV (bOPV) containing types 1 and 3; monovalent OPV (mOPV) for types 1 and 3. Type 2 mOPV has also been developed recently and is important for use in stockpiles available for potential outbreak control in the posteradication era.

Although seroconversion rates to tOPV approach 100% in developed countries against all 3 serotypes, developing countries generally have much lower rates of detectable antibodies after vaccination with 3 doses of tOPV particularly to types 1 and 3. An analysis of seroconversion studies found an average rate of only 73% to type 1 and 70% to type 3.[12] Data suggest that the type 2 component in OPV as well as ubiquitous enteric viruses present in developing countries interfere with responses to types 1 and 3.[12] The inferior immunogenicity in developing countries can be overcome by additional doses (sometimes more than 10) of OPV, which lead to population immunity levels exceeding herd immunity thresholds for stopping transmission. In addition, OPV is sensitive to heat and must be transported in an intact cold chain, which proves difficult in rural and hard-to-reach areas, locations where the last reservoirs of WPV remain.

Thus far, OPV has been the mainstay of polio eradication. The live vaccine is inexpensive (less than 15¢ per dose through the United Nations Children's Fund), simple to administer (does not require a trained health worker or produce sharps waste), and induces intestinal mucosal immunity in reducing transmission in settings in which fecal-oral transmission predominates. A systematic review of mucosal immunity of polio vaccines found that individuals vaccinated with OPV were protected against shedding of poliovirus in stool samples collected after challenge (an indicator of induction of intestinal mucosal immunity) compared with unvaccinated individuals (odds ratio, 0.13; 95% confidence interval, 0.08–0.24).[13] In contrast, the proportion of IPV recipients who shed after an OPV challenge is not different than naive persons receiving OPV for the first time (see later for further discussion of IPV).

Risks of Oral Poliovirus Vaccine
Vaccine-associated paralytic polio During the replication process, the Sabin strains of OPV can mutate and rarely revert to neurovirulent variants causing paralysis clinically indistinguishable from that caused by WPV.[14] Vaccine-associated paralytic polio (VAPP) causes paralysis in OPV recipients and close contacts. In a review of epidemiology and burden, the global risk of VAPP was determined to be 4.7 cases per million births or approximately 500 cases of VAPP estimated globally, per year, with 90% estimated to occur in low- and lower-middle-income countries.[15] About 26% to 31% of VAPP cases were associated with the type 2 component of tOPV.[15]

Circulating vaccine-derived poliovirus Vaccine virus can rarely mutate and regain both the neurovirulence and transmissibility properties of WPVs, causing outbreaks of polio. When prolonged replication of the vaccine virus takes place (isolates having >1% divergence [0.6% for type 2] from the original OPV strain), the virus is considered a VDPV.[3] VDPVs are grouped into 1 of 3 categories: (1) immunodeficient VDPVs isolated from individuals with B-cell immunodeficiency who maintain chronic infection after vaccination with OPV, (2) cVDPVs requiring evidence of person-to-person transmission in the community (eg, cluster of $\geq$2 AFP cases), and (3) ambiguous VDPVs (aVDPVs), which do not belong to the previous categories.[3]

The largest risk factor for generation of cVDPVs is low overall population immunity allowing vaccine viruses to mutate and spread within a susceptible population.[16,17] cVDPV outbreaks have occurred in areas with complex challenges, such as those with insecurity, poor infrastructure, and low immunization coverage, and can easily spread beyond borders, causing outbreaks and sporadic cases elsewhere. Outbreaks in Pakistan, Afghanistan, Nigeria, and Somalia have occurred in conjunction with WPV outbreaks in areas where groups of children remain unvaccinated because of conflict and poor access. Repeated SIAs using OPV containing the parent Sabin strain of the strain causing the outbreak have been shown to stop cVDPV outbreaks.[18]

Inactivated Poliovirus Vaccine

The current IPV formulation contains 40-8-32 D-Antigen units for poliovirus types 1, 2, and 3, respectively, and is available in stand-alone vaccine or as multivalent presentations.[19] Made from selected WPV strains grown in Vero cell culture or human diploid cells, IPV establishes a strong immune response in recipients. Nearly 100% seroconversion rates and high antibody titers to all 3 serotypes are seen after 3 doses and greater than 90% seroconversion rates after 2 doses when administered after 8 weeks of age.[20] Immunogenicity depends on the number of doses as well as the age of administration because of interference of maternal antibodies in infants. In a study in Puerto Rico comparing US schedules (2, 4, and 6 months) with WHO's Expanded Programme on Immunization (EPI) schedules (6, 10, and 14 weeks), seroconversion rates were lower for types 1 and 2 in the EPI schedule study arm, whereby maternal antibody levels were higher.[21]

In another study in Cuba, 63% of infants seroconverted to type 2 after a single dose of IPV when administered at 4 months of age.[22] Among those who did not seroconvert after 1 dose of IPV, 98% had a priming response to a subsequent dose of IPV, that is, they developed significant antibody responses within 7 days of subsequent exposure to IPV.[22] Although seroconversion is associated with protection from paralysis, questions remain as to whether persons who are primed are protected from disease (ie, can antibody be made quickly enough after exposure to provide protection). Experience in Hungary, which had a major problem with VAPP, showed that VAPP was eliminated when the country chose a sequential IPV/OPV schedule with 1 dose of IPV followed by OPV, suggesting priming is protective.[23] Conversely, an outbreak of WPV1 in Senegal was associated with 36% effectiveness after 1 dose and 89% effectiveness after 2 doses, a finding more compatible with the need to seroconvert to assure protection.[24]

Studies have shown neutralizing antibodies against poliovirus to persist for at least 5 years in all vaccine recipients after a primary immunization series of 3 to 4 doses.[25,26] Antibody concentration may decline with time in some people, although no association has been seen with antibody less than detectable levels and increased susceptibility to paralytic disease.[27] As all high-income countries administer 3 or more doses, the precise duration of immunity for 1 or 2 doses of IPV remains less understood.[27]

Concerns raised with Inactivated Poliovirus Vaccine

IPV, whether give alone or with other vaccines, is considered to be safe and has not been causally associated with any serious adverse events.[27] The high immunogenicity provided by IPV leads to high levels of individual protection against paralysis in the recipient. However, IPV is less effective in inducing intestinal mucosal immunity than OPV among previously unvaccinated individuals, although quantity and duration of shedding may be reduced.[13] For this reason, IPV does not provide the same amount of community protection against transmission that OPV does. In addition, IPV is more expensive than OPV, with negotiated costs for developing countries of $1 or more per dose when compared with 15¢ for a dose of OPV. IPV, a vaccine administered intramuscularly, requires trained health workers and produces sharps waste. As IPV is produced from WPV strains, there is a risk of accidental release during production, as has happened in The Netherlands in 1992 and Belgium in 2014.[28,29] Because a release in a developing country with crowding, poor hygiene, and sanitation is more risky than in an industrialized country, IPV manufacture from WPV strains is limited to a few developed countries, limiting global production capacity.

Israel (and the WHO European Region) was certified polio free in 2002. Israel initiated an IPV-only schedule in 2005 and also has an extensive environmental surveillance system to detect viruses. In early February 2013, WPV1 was isolated indicating an introduction into the Southern districts, although no paralytic polio cases were detected.[30] Officials responded with intensified environmental surveillance, a bOPV SIA, and an addition of 1 dose of bOPV back into the routine immunization schedule.[30] WPV circulation took place for more than 1 year, with termination of transmission in March of 2014. The experience alerted the public health community to the continued need for OPV in areas where fecal-oral spread of wild viruses is predominant, the value of environmental surveillance in addition to AFP surveillance in countries at particular risk, and the need for mOPV stockpiles in the posteradication era in case wild viruses are reintroduced.[31]

In contrast, Yogyakarta, Indonesia, switched from OPV to only IPV in 2007. In this experience, no cVDPVs emerged. Thus, IPV may be more effective in preventing the emergence of cVDPVs because of the lower force of infection of polio vaccine viruses than wild viruses versus curtailing transmission of WPVs or existing cVDPVs.[32] In addition, IPV alone has eliminated polio in Nordic countries and other industrialized countries that have switched to only IPV, where oral-to-oral transmission is thought to be the predominant mode of transmission. With the exception of Israel, all these countries have maintained a WPV-free status.[33]

USING ORAL AND INACTIVATED POLIOVIRUS VACCINES TOGETHER

Administration of IPV before OPV has been shown to prevent the incidence of VAPP in some areas, a schedule that theoretically uses the humoral and mucosal strengths of both vaccines.[27] Effective reduction in VAPP after introduction of IPV/OPV sequential schedules has been seen in Denmark[34] (3 doses of IPV followed by 3 doses of OPV), Hungary[23] (1 dose of IPV followed by 3 doses of OPV), and the United States[35] (2 doses of IPV followed by 2 doses of OPV).

Studies examining IPV use in children previously vaccinated with tOPV have suggested that IPV is effective at closing immunity gaps, especially for type 2 poliovirus.[36,37] In fact, a single dose of IPV in infants and children previously vaccinated with multiple doses of OPV reduced the prevalence of shedding by 39% to 76% and boosted mucosal immunity for types 1 and 3 after OPV challenge compared with no vaccination.[38,39] A birth dose of OPV allows for induction of mucosal immunity before infants are exposed to enteric pathogens and increases seroconversion rates.[27]

Simultaneous use of OPV and IPV in developing countries has shown induction of high antibody responses to all 3 poliovirus types.[27] In a 3-country study, concomitant administration of OPV and IPV at 6, 10, and 14 weeks after a birth dose of OPV yielded the highest seroconversion rates in Oman and The Gambia when compared with OPV only given at the same schedule. The third country, Thailand, illustrated similar seroconversion rates in both groups.[40]

ENDGAME STRATEGY AND TIMELINE

Despite the significant gains made in reduction of the number of polio cases due to OPV, the rare adverse events including VAPP and VDPVs require the phased withdrawal of all OPV use in the final stage of the eradication process.[41] The 2013–18 Eradication and Endgame Strategic Plan[41] describes complete interruption of transmission and elimination of all polio disease, which includes WPV, VDPVs, and VAPP, using the available tools of OPV and IPV followed by withdrawal of OPV use.

In recent years, the serotype profile of cVDPVs has shifted, with type 2 related cVDPVs representing a larger proportion of all cVDPV cases (97% of the 628 cases of cVDPV from 2006–2013).[18] This trend can be seen in **Fig. 2** and is thought to be due to increased use of bOPV in campaigns in recent years, leading to reduced population immunity to type 2, a risk factor for cVDPV emergence.[42,43] In addition, type 2 WPV seems to have been eradicated with the last naturally occurring case detected in 1999. Because type 2 also causes a proportion of VAPP cases, type 2 vaccine virus is causing harm and potentially doing little good. Thus, the strategic plan calls for global, synchronized replacement of tOPV with bOPV after prior introduction of at least 1 dose of IPV into routine immunization schedules in all 125 countries using OPV only.[41] Introduction of IPV will ensure that a proportion of the population is protected against type 2 polio, boost immunity to types 1 and 3, and mitigate other risks associated with the switch.

After IPV introduction, the globally synchronized switch is scheduled to occur in April 2016. WHO will assess global readiness and monitor the absence of all persistent cVDPV2s globally as a precondition for implementing the switch. These events represent a public health effort unprecedented in time and scope and will require coordination and partnership across many global, national, and local organizations as well as public-private partnership.

CHALLENGES AND OPPORTUNITIES

India, one of the last countries to eradicate smallpox, was believed by some to be a near-impossible location for the eradication of polio because of high population density, poor sanitation, weak immunization systems, remote villages, and massive

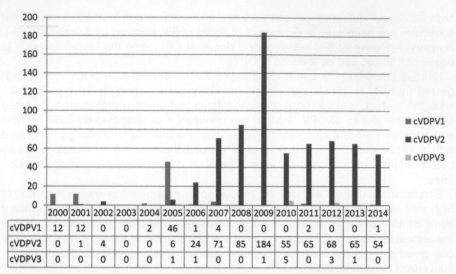

	2000	2001	2002	2003	2004	2005	2006	2007	2008	2009	2010	2011	2012	2013	2014
cVDPV1	12	12	0	0	2	46	1	4	0	0	0	2	0	0	1
cVDPV2	0	1	4	0	0	6	24	71	85	184	55	65	68	65	54
cVDPV3	0	0	0	0	0	1	1	0	0	1	5	0	3	1	0

Fig. 2. Reported paralytic cases of cVDPV by type worldwide, 2000–14 (as of July 28, 2015). (*Adapted from* Patel M, Zipursky S, Orenstein W, et al. Polio endgame: the global introduction of inactivated polio vaccine. Expert Rev Vaccines 2015;14(5):752; with permission; and *Data from* http://www.polioeradication.org/Dataandmonitoring/Poliothisweek/Circulatingvaccinederivedpoliovirus.aspx. Accessed July 30, 2015.)

migrant populations. But as a result of strong ownership and resource investments from the local to national level, accountability, and international partnerships, India (and the entire South-East Asian region) was certified polio free by WHO in March 2014.[44,45] Important lessons learned from India's exceptional polio eradication effort include development of detailed plans to maintain high coverage in SIAs, close monitoring and supervision, robust communication strategies, and research and innovation to overcome operational barriers to ensure every child is vaccinated.[46]

Pakistan, on the other hand, remains the engine of WPV transmission. In 2014, 85% of WPV cases seen worldwide were detected in Pakistan and many cases in neighboring Afghanistan were imported across the border from Pakistan.[8] For years after mid-2012 when local authorities banned polio vaccination, nearly 350,000 children in some districts of the Federally Administered Tribal Areas had not received polio vaccine during SIAs.[47] That number has since decreased to less than 50,000.[48] In other areas of Pakistan, polio workers (often women) have been attacked and killed. Although great strides have been made in the last year, until all children in conflict-affected areas can be reached with vaccine, Pakistan remains a major challenge for interruption of WPV. Substantial progress has been made in the African region as Nigeria should soon be removed from the list of endemic countries (ie, countries which have never interrupted transmission of indigenous strains of poliovirus).

POSTERADICATION RISKS AND MITIGATION

As WPV cases continue to decrease and the world inches closer to polio eradication, considerations of late-stage risks are essential. Reintroduction of WPV and release from manufacturers or laboratories are of ultimate concern. The endgame plan calls for appropriate handling and containment of all infectious poliovirus stocks from biomedical facilities to ensure that WPV cannot be transmitted to an increasingly

Table 3
Ongoing research on current and future tools for polio eradication

Research Question/Tool	Importance	Status
Current tools		
Combination schedules of IPV and OPV	Understand role of IPV and bOPV when used together in recommended schedules in developing countries	Immunogenicity (humoral and intestinal) of ≥1 IPV dose combined with bOPV in 6–10–14 wk mixed schedules (Colombia-Dominican Republic-Guatemala-Panama, India, Bangladesh) Immunogenicity (humoral and intestinal) of IPV → bOPV in 2-4-6 mo sequential regimen (Chile) Duration of protection of boosting of intestinal immunity induced by IPV in OPV primed populations (India)
Fractional doses of IPV	Reduced cost	Immunogenicity with fractional IPV doses via ID route (The Gambia, Bangladesh)
New tools		
Immunogenicity of monovalent IPV-2 (m-IPV2)	Improved humoral and intestinal immunogenicity Reduced cost with 1 dose of m-IPV2	Phase I (Belgium) study on safety completed Phase II (Panama) study underway to evaluate safety and immunogenicity
Immunogenicity of IPV adjuvants	Reduced cost Increased supply Potential for enhanced mucosal immunity	Clinical studies being planned to evaluate potential for aluminum salts adjuvants and for dmLT (double-mutant heat-labile enterotoxin) adjuvants for IPV
Feasibility of novel routes of administration	Operational advantages Potential for use in SIAs Concomitant use with other vaccines	Studies in humans being planned or implemented to evaluate impact of IM (Intramuscular) and ID (Intradermal) delivery of IPV through use of disposable jet injectors, microneedle patch, and other novel delivery techniques
Development of genetically stable OPV and attenuated IPV seed strains	Potential use in outbreak control (reduced risk of VDPVs and VAPP) or in routine immunization if IPV is considered inadequate in reducing transmission risk Further attenuated and less infectious seed strains for safe IPV manufacture	In preclinical development or planning phase
Immunogenicity with Sabin IPV	Minimize risk of reintroduction of WPV from IPV manufacturing facilities	Sabin IPV has been licensed in Japan Efficacy and feasibility of large-scale production are currently being evaluated

Adapted from Bandyopadhyay AS, Garon J, Seib K, et al. Polio vaccination: past, present and future. Future Microbiol 2015;801–2. http://dx.doi.org/10.2217/fmb.15.19.

susceptible community.[41] Shedding of VDPV among adults and children with primary B-cell immunodeficiency constitutes a long-term risk, as those individuals have been shown to shed virus for up to several years after administration of OPV, a consideration as long as OPV vaccination continues.[49]

The cost for maintenance of current levels of vaccination, program implementation, surveillance and laboratory capacity, and outbreak response are estimated to be $5.5 billion dollars for current global strategic plan.[41] The cost of abandoning global eradication efforts completely is substantial in terms of program costs, treatment costs, and human lives lost. Estimated incremental net benefits of the GPEI between 1988 and 2035 amount to approximately $40 billion to $50 billion saved through eradication efforts.[50] Letting the pressure off now is expected to result in skyrocketing numbers of cases. GPEI is the single largest internationally coordinated public health effort in history and there is strong economic justification for finishing the job completely.[50]

RESEARCH NEEDS

These final stages of the polio eradication endgame have revealed unique challenges to eliminating the disease from areas with the last reservoirs of virus, leading to innovation in vaccine technology and delivery. At this stage in the polio endgame, focus is being placed on new innovations such as technology to help achieve lower-cost IPV, strategies to make vaccine manufacture safer, and operational advances to make vaccine administration simpler.[43] Specifics on areas of research on OPV and IPV can be seen in **Table 3**.[51]

ROLE OF NORTH AMERICAN PHYSICIANS

Even though naturally occurring paralytic poliomyelitis has not been seen in the United States since 1979, physicians play an important role in the global polio eradication effort. Current Advisory Committee on Immunization Practices recommendations for routine polio immunization include 4 doses of IPV to be given at ages 2, 4, and 6 to 18 months and 4 to 6 years.[52] Physicians should ensure that all patients receive routine childhood polio immunization and that travelers are vaccinated with an additional dose of IPV if they will be visiting a country with polio infection.[10] New International Health Regulations require proof of vaccination of a dose of polio vaccine when leaving a country with polio infection (long-term travelers staying for >4 weeks). The dose should be given at least 4 weeks and no more than 12 months before departure.[9]

Although diagnosis of poliomyelitis in the United States is rare, physicians should suspect polio in a patient who presents with a clinically compatible case. There may not be a history of travel to a polio endemic or epidemic country as the transmitting infection could be subclinical. At least 2 stool samples should be collected, 24 hours apart, ideally within 14 days of the onset of paralysis. A single case of suspected paralytic polio demands immediate attention. Timely notification of state health department and CDC is critical. Finally, US physicians should advocate for and support introduction of IPV in developing countries as well as US government support for the overall initiative. As long as WPV exists anywhere, risk of importation exists everywhere.[53]

REFERENCES

1. Hinman AR, Koplan JP, Orenstein WA, et al. Live or inactivated poliomyelitis vaccine: an analysis of benefits and risks. Am J Public Health 1988;78(3):291–5.

2. Cochi SL, Dowdle WR. Disease eradication in the 21st century: implications for global health. Cambridge (MA): MIT Press Books; 2011. Available at: http://mitpress.mit.edu/books/disease-eradication-21st-century. Accessed May 10, 2015.
3. Poliomyelitis (Polio). In World Health Organization, International travel and health. 2014. Available at http://www.who.int/ith/diseases/polio/en/. Accessed December 22, 2014.
4. WHO | Poliomyelitis (Polio). WHO. Available at: http://www.who.int/ith/diseases/polio/en/. Accessed December 22, 2014.
5. Wiechers D. Electrophysiology of acute polio revisited. Ann N Y Acad Sci 1995; 753(1):111–9.
6. Sutter RW, Kew OM, Cochi SL, et al. 28-Poliovirus vaccine—live, Table 28–2: causes and differential diagnosis of acute flaccid paralysis. In: Plotkin SA, Orenstein WA, Offit PA, editors. Vaccines (sixth edition). London: W.B. Saunders; 2013. p. 603. Available at: http://www.sciencedirect.com/science/article/pii/B9781455700905000355.
7. Jorba J, Campagnoli R, De L, et al. Calibration of multiple poliovirus molecular clocks covering an extended evolutionary range. J Virol 2008;82(9):4429–40.
8. The Global Polio Eradication Initiative. Data Monit. 2015. Available at: http://www.polioeradication.org/Dataandmonitoring.aspx. Accessed March 27, 2015.
9. WHO | WHO statement on the meeting of the International Health Regulations Emergency Committee concerning the international spread of wild poliovirus. WHO. Available at: http://www.who.int/mediacentre/news/statements/2014/polio-20140505/en/. Accessed May 14, 2014.
10. Wallace GS, Seward JF, Pallansch MA, et al, Centers for Disease Control and Prevention. Interim CDC guidance for polio vaccination for travel to and from countries affected by wild poliovirus. MMWR Morb Mortal Wkly Rep 2014;63(27): 591–4. Available at: http://www.cdc.gov/mmwr/preview/mmwrhtml/mm6327a4.htm?s_cid=mm6327a4_w. Accessed January 8, 2015.
11. Porter KA, Diop OM, Burns CC, et al. Tracking progress toward polio eradication—worldwide, 2013–2014. MMWR Morb Mortal Wkly Rep 2015;64(15): 415–20. Available at: http://www.cdc.gov/mmwr/preview/mmwrhtml/mm6415a4.htm?s_cid=mm6415a4_w. Accessed April 23, 2015.
12. Patriarca PA, Wright PF, John TJ. Factors affecting the immunogenicity of oral poliovirus vaccine in developing countries: review. Rev Infect Dis 1991;13(5):926–39.
13. Hird TR, Grassly NC. Systematic review of mucosal immunity induced by oral and inactivated poliovirus vaccines against virus shedding following oral poliovirus challenge. PLoS Pathog 2012;8(4):e1002599.
14. Dowdle WR, De Gourville E, Kew OM, et al. Polio eradication: the OPV paradox. Rev Med Virol 2003;13(5):277–91.
15. Platt LR, Estívariz CF, Sutter RW. Vaccine-associated paralytic poliomyelitis: a review of the epidemiology and estimation of the global burden. J Infect Dis 2014; 210(Suppl 1):S380–9.
16. Kew O, Morris-Glasgow V, Landaverde M, et al. Outbreak of poliomyelitis in Hispaniola associated with circulating type 1 vaccine-derived poliovirus. Science 2002;296(5566):356–9.
17. Estívariz CF, Watkins MA, Handoko D, et al. A large vaccine-derived poliovirus outbreak on Madura Island—Indonesia, 2005. J Infect Dis 2008;197(3):347–54.
18. Update on vaccine-derived polioviruses—worldwide, July 2012–December 2013. Centers for Disease Control and Prevention. Available at: http://www.cdc.gov/mmwr/preview/mmwrhtml/mm6311a5.htm. Accessed February 3, 2015.

19. Vidor E. 27-Poliovirus vaccine-inactivated. In: Plotkin SA, Orenstein WA, Offit PA, editors. Vaccines (sixth edition). Philadelphia: Elsevier/Saunders; 2013. p. 573–97.
20. Estivariz CF, Pallansch MA, Anand A, et al. Poliovirus vaccination options for achieving eradication and securing the endgame. Curr Opin Virol 2013;3(3): 309–15.
21. Dayan GH, Thorley M, Yamamura Y, et al. Serologic response to inactivated poliovirus vaccine: a randomized clinical trial comparing 2 vaccination schedules in Puerto Rico. J Infect Dis 2007;195(1):12–20.
22. Resik S, Tejeda A, Sutter RW, et al. Priming after a fractional dose of inactivated poliovirus vaccine. N Engl J Med 2013;368(5):416–24.
23. Dömök I. Experiences associated with the use of live poliovirus vaccine in Hungary, 1959–1982. Rev Infect Dis 1984;6(Suppl 2):S413–8.
24. Robertson SE, Traverso HP, Drucker JA, et al. Clinical efficacy of a new, enhanced-potency, inactivated poliovirus vaccine. Lancet 1988;1(8591):897–9.
25. Carlsson R-M, Claesson BA, Fagerlund E, et al. Antibody persistence in five-year-old children who received a pentavalent combination vaccine in infancy. Pediatr Infect Dis J 2002;21(6):535–41.
26. Langue J, Matisse N, Pacoret P, et al. Persistence of antibodies at 5–6 years of age for children who had received a primary series vaccination with a pentavalent whole-cell pertussis vaccine and a first booster with a pentavalent acellular pertussis vaccine: immunogenicity and tolerance of second booster with a tetravalent acellular vaccine at 5–6 years of age. Vaccine 2004;22(11–12):1406–14.
27. Weekly Epidemiological Record. Polio vaccines: who position paper, January 2014. World Health Organization; 2014. p. 73–92. Available at: http://www.who.int/wer/2014/wer8909.pdf?ua=1. Accessed December 22, 2014.
28. Mulders MN, Reimerink JHJ, Koopmans MPG, et al. Genetic analysis of wild-type poliovirus importation into the Netherlands (1979–1995). J Infect Dis 1997;176(3): 617–24.
29. Accidental release of 45 litres of concentrated live polio virus solution into the environment - Belgium. European Centre for Disease Prevention and Control. 2014. Available at: http://ecdc.europa.eu/en/publications/Publications/communicable-disease-threats-report-13-sep-2014.pdf. Accessed May 9, 2015.
30. Anis E, Kopel E, Singer S, et al. Insidious reintroduction of wild poliovirus into Israel, 2013. Euro Surveill 2013;18(38):1–5. Available at: http://www.ncbi.nlm.nih.gov/pubmed/24084337.
31. Kopel E, Kaliner E, Grotto I. Lessons from a public health emergency—importation of wild poliovirus to Israel. N Engl J Med 2014;371(11):981–3.
32. Wahjuhono G, Revolusiana, Widhiastuti D, et al. Switch from oral to inactivated poliovirus vaccine in Yogyakarta province, Indonesia: summary of coverage, immunity, and environmental surveillance. J Infect Dis 2014;210(Suppl 1):S347–52.
33. Bonnet M-C, Dutta A. Worldwide experience with inactivated poliovirus vaccine. Vaccine 2008;26(39):4978–83.
34. Von Magnus H, Petersen I. Vaccination with inactivated poliovirus vaccine and oral poliovirus vaccine in Denmark. Rev Infect Dis 1984;6(Suppl 2):S471–4.
35. Alexander L, Seward JF, Santibanez TA, et al. Vaccine policy changes and epidemiology of poliomyelitis in the united states. JAMA 2004;292(14):1696–701.
36. Hanlon P, Hanlon L, Marsh V, et al. Serological comparisons of approaches to polio vaccination in The Gambia. Lancet 1987;1(8536):800–1.
37. Moriniere BJ, Van Loon FPL, Rhodes PH, et al. Immunogenicity of a supplemental dose of oral versus inactivated poliovirus vaccine. The Lancet 1993;341(8860): 1545–50.

38. John J, Giri S, Karthikeyan AS, et al. Effect of a single inactivated poliovirus vaccine dose on intestinal immunity against poliovirus in children previously given oral vaccine: an open-label, randomised controlled trial. The Lancet 2014; 384(9953):1505–12.
39. Jafari H, Deshpande JM, Sutter RW, et al. Efficacy of inactivated poliovirus vaccine in India. Science 2014;345(6199):922–5.
40. Combined immunization of infants with oral and inactivated poliovirus vaccines: results of a randomized trial in The Gambia, Oman, and Thailand. WHO Collaborative Study Group on Oral and Inactivated Poliovirus Vaccines. Bull World Health Organ 1996;74(3):253–68.
41. Global Polio Eradication Initiative. Polio Eradication & Endgame Strategic Plan 2013-2018. 2013. Available at: http://www.polioeradication.org/Portals/0/Document/Resources/StrategyWork/PEESP_EN_US.pdf. Accessed May 16, 2015.
42. Global Polio Eradication Initiative. Circulating vaccine-derived poliovirus 2000-2013. 2013. Available at: http://www.polioeradication.org/Dataandmonitoring/Poliothisweek/Circulatingvaccinederivedpoliovirus.aspx. Accessed March 5, 2015.
43. Patel M, Zipursky S, Orenstein W, et al. Polio endgame: the global introduction of inactivated polio vaccine. Expert Rev Vaccines 2015;14(5):749–62.
44. SEARO | India three years polio-free. SEARO. Available at: http://www.searo.who.int/mediacentre/features/2014/sea-polio/en/. Accessed February 26, 2015.
45. SEARO | WHO South-East Asia Region certified polio-free. SEARO. Available at: http://www.searo.who.int/mediacentre/releases/2014/pr1569/en/. Accessed February 26, 2015.
46. Polio-free certification and lessons learned—South-East Asia region, March 2014. Available at: http://www.cdc.gov/mmwr/preview/mmwrhtml/mm6342a2.htm. Accessed February 26, 2015.
47. Alexander JP, Zubair M, Khan M, et al. Progress and peril: poliomyelitis eradication efforts in Pakistan, 1994–2013. J Infect Dis 2014;210(Suppl 1):S152–61.
48. WHO | Statement on the 5th IHR Emergency Committee meeting regarding the international spread of wild poliovirus. WHO. Available at: http://who.int/mediacentre/news/statements/2015/polio-5th-statement/en/. Accessed May 15, 2015.
49. Grassly NC. The final stages of the global eradication of poliomyelitis. Philos Trans R Soc Lond B Biol Sci 2013;368(1623):20120140.
50. Duintjer Tebbens RJ, Pallansch MA, Cochi SL, et al. Economic analysis of the global polio eradication initiative. Vaccine 2010;29(2):334–43.
51. Bandyopadhyay AS, Garon J, Seib K, et al. Polio vaccination: past, present and future. Future Microbiol 2015;10:791–808.
52. Vaccines: ACIP vaccine recommendations - polio - CDC. Available at: http://www.cdc.gov/vaccines/hcp/acip-recs/vacc-specific/polio.html. Accessed October 14, 2014.
53. Mundel T, Orenstein WA. No country is safe without global eradication of poliomyelitis. N Engl J Med 2013;369(21):2045–6.

The Changing Epidemiology of Meningococcal Disease

 CrossMark

Amanda Cohn, MD[a],*, Jessica MacNeil, MPH[b]

KEYWORDS

• *Neisseria meningitidis* • Meningococcal disease • Vaccination

KEY POINTS

• The incidence of meningococcal disease is currently at an historic low in the United States, but prevention remains a priority because of the devastating outcomes and risk for outbreaks.

• Vaccines are available to protect against all major serogroups of *Neisseria meningitidis* circulating in the United States. These vaccines are recommended routinely for persons at increased risk for disease. In addition, adolescents are routinely recommended to receive quadrivalent meningococcal conjugate vaccine (MenACWY) starting at age 11 years.

• Although vaccination has virtually eliminated serogroup A meningococcal outbreaks from the Meningitis Belt of Africa and reduced the incidence of serogroup C disease around the world, eradication of *N meningitidis* will unlikely be achieved by currently available vaccines because of the continued carriage and transmission of nonencapsulated organisms, which is not affected by the use of polysaccharide vaccines.

INTRODUCTION

Neisseria meningitidis is a gram-negative, encapsulated diplococcus that exclusively infects humans. Twelve distinct serogroups have been identified based on their capsular polysaccharide, with serogroups A, B, C, W, and Y accounting for nearly all disease. In the United States, serogroup B accounts for approximately 65% of infant meningococcal disease, while serogroups C and Y caused the majority of disease in adolescents prior to routine vaccination, and serogroup Y predominates in the elderly.[1]

[a] Immunization Services Division, National Center for Immunization and Respiratory Diseases, Centers for Disease Control and Prevention, Atlanta, GA, USA; [b] Bacterial Diseases Division, National Center for Immunization and Respiratory Diseases, Centers for Disease Control and Prevention, Atlanta, GA, USA
* Corresponding author.
E-mail address: anc0@cdc.gov

Infect Dis Clin N Am 29 (2015) 667–677
http://dx.doi.org/10.1016/j.idc.2015.08.002
0891-5520/15/$ – see front matter Published by Elsevier Inc.

id.theclinics.com

N meningitidis is a transient commensal of the human nasopharynx. Nasopharyngeal carriage rates are highest in adolescents and young adults, who serve as reservoirs for transmission of *N meningitidis*.[2] Acquisition of the organism and colonization of the nasopharynx is necessary for the development of disease, but not sufficient. In most cases carriage is an immunizing event, resulting in protective antibodies that prevent disease.

meningococcal disease is a rare but devastating infectious disease in the United States. Disease incidence is at an historic low, but several large outbreaks of serogroup B meningococcal disease have occurred on college campuses since 2008. The current historically low incidence of meningococcal disease in the United States is juxtaposed with the rapid onset of disease, high case fatality, and substantial long-term sequelae among survivors, and the potential for outbreaks, making decisions about use of meningococcal vaccines challenging.

Quadrivalent meningococcal conjugate vaccines (MenACWY) have been licensed in the United States since 2005 and are recommended for routine use among adolescents aged 11 through 18 years.[3] Before licensure and use of these vaccines, 75% of disease in persons aged 11 years or older was caused by serogroups C, Y, or W.[4] Among adolescents, the remainder of disease is caused by serogroup B, for which 2 vaccines were licensed in 2014 and 2015. Persons at increased risk for meningococcal disease are routinely recommended to receive MenACWY and serogroup B meningococcal (MenB) vaccine.[5] Recommendations for use of MenB vaccines in adolescents not at increased risk are not yet available.

THE DISEASE AS CANDIDATE FOR ERADICATION

With currently available prevention tools, *N meningitidis* is not a candidate for eradication because of the commensal nature of the bacteria in the nasopharynx. Nonencapsulated *Neisseria* organisms are transmitted and have multiple genetic mechanisms to alter their antigenic profile, including capsular switching.[6] An example of capsular switching is the serogroup W strain that caused a large outbreak in 2000 among Hajj pilgrims. This clone spread globally and caused infection in multiple geographic locations, with a large outbreak in the Meningitis Belt of Africa during 2001 to 2002. The Hajj clone was genetically associated with strains that typically cause serogroup C disease.[7]

Capsular replacement after vaccination against 1 or more serogroups is another concern. In the United Kingdom there was no evidence of capsule replacement after vaccine implementation, although several years after the introduction of MenC vaccine, serogroups W and Y disease have been increasing.[8,9] However, the incidence of serogroups W and Y disease is still considerably lower than the incidence of serogroup C disease before vaccination. There is no evidence of capsular replacement after MenACWY introduction in the United States; serogroup B disease in the United States has continued to decline in incidence, along with serogroups C and Y.[3]

Although the bacteria as a whole cannot be eradicated, it is possible to drastically reduce transmission of specific clones causing hyperendemic disease or outbreaks in defined geographic areas. There have been several recent examples of this, including the elimination of a clonal serogroup C strain causing increased rates of disease in the United Kingdom with the introduction of a MenC conjugate vaccine, and the elimination of serogroup A epidemics in Africa with MenA conjugate vaccine.[10–12] In both of these examples, the countries implemented mass vaccination programs in target age groups and achieved high coverage rapidly. In the United Kingdom, there was no evidence of serogroup replacement of the hyperendemic clonal strain.

However, in 2014 and 2015, Nigeria and Niger experienced large serogroup C outbreaks, the latter outbreak in Niger causing more than 5000 cases in less than 6 months.[13] This highlights the challenges of eliminating outbreaks of meningococcal disease entirely.

CLINICAL ASPECTS

Initial manifestation can be nonspecific and difficult to distinguish from other infections such as influenza, but typically is abrupt, with fever, limb pain, and headache (2015 Red Book). The early rash may be maculopapular or petechial and can be indistinguishable from other viral rashes, but as disease progresses more classic purpura can develop (2015 Red Book).

Invasive disease typically results in meningitis (50% of cases) or bacteremia (30%–40%). Fulminant meningococcemia with purpura and refractory septic shock occurs in approximately 20% of patients with bacteremia, and results from rapid proliferation of meningococci in the blood (**Fig. 1**). Other localized infections including pneumonia and septic arthritis present less commonly. Bloodstream infection can occur with or without other localized infection. Long-term sequelae including limb loss, hearing loss, skin scarring, and neurologic deficits occur in approximately 11% to 19% of cases. The overall case fatality is approximately 10% to 15%, and is as high as 25% to 30% in patients with meningococcemia.[14]

Cultures of the blood and cerebrospinal fluid are critical to identify *N meningitidis* as the causative organism. For suspected cases that are culture negative, which can occur especially if the cultures are taken after the first dose of antimicrobial therapy, detection of *N meningitidis*–specific nucleic acid by a validated polymerase chain reaction can confirm a diagnosis (available at http://wwwn.cdc.gov/nndss/conditions/meningococcal-disease/case-definition/2015/). All suspected cases should be treated with an extended-spectrum cephalosporin, such as ceftriaxone plus vancomycin, until organisms with high penicillin resistance, such as *Streptococcus pneumoniae*, are ruled out. Once the diagnosis is established, treatment with penicillin G, ampicillin, or an extended-spectrum cephalosporin is recommended (2015 Red Book). Antimicrobial resistance testing is not routinely recommended, but some experts do recommend testing before changing to penicillin G. Fortunately, strains of *N meningitidis* in the United States are rarely found to be resistant to the commonly

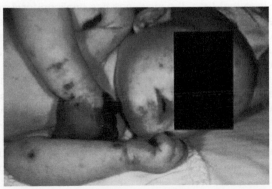

Fig. 1. A 4-month-old female with gangrene of hands caused by meningococcemia. (*Courtesy of* CDC Public Health Image Library. CDC/ Mr. Gust.)

used antimicrobials.[15] Intermediate penicillin susceptibility is reported, but the clinical significance of these strains on patient outcomes is unknown.

All suspected cases of meningococcal disease should be reported to the local health department. Antimicrobial chemoprophylaxis of close contacts is important to prevent secondary cases. The Centers for Disease Control and Prevention (CDC) define close contacts as (1) household members, (2) child-care center or preschool contacts, and (3) anyone with unprotected exposure to the patient's respiratory secretions or aerosols, or other exposures indicating close or intimate contact (eg, kissing, mouth-to-mouth resuscitation, endotracheal tube management) in the 7 days before symptom onset (http://www.cdc.gov/meningococcal/downloads/interim-guidance. pdf). Rifampin, ciprofloxacin, and ceftriaxone are 90% to 95% effective in reducing nasopharyngeal carriage of N meningitidis and are all acceptable antimicrobial agents for chemoprophylaxis.[3] For prevention of additional cases during an outbreak, vaccination is the primary strategy, and mass chemoprophylaxis is generally not recommended. However, mass chemoprophylaxis may be considered as an interim measure to temporarily reduce meningococcal carriage and transmission in the population in the period before potential protection from vaccination can be achieved (http://www.cdc.gov/meningococcal/downloads/interim-guidance.pdf). There are limited data regarding the use of currently recommended antimicrobials and whether additional cases are prevented by mass chemoprophylaxis.

EPIDEMIOLOGY

The incidence of meningococcal disease is highest in sub-Saharan Africa where, before broad introduction of a serogroup A conjugate vaccine, incidence ranged from 10 to 25 per 100,000 during nonepidemic periods and up to 1000 per 100,000 during epidemic years.[16] The incidence in Canada, the United States, and Europe varies substantially by country, ranging from 0.18 per 100,000 to 3 per 100,000 persons per year.[16] In industrialized countries the incidence of meningococcal disease varies by age, with infants younger than 1 year at greatest risk, followed by a second peak in incidence observed among adolescents (**Fig. 2**).[1] However, cases occur in all age groups, making the development of vaccination strategies challenging.

In the United States, the incidence of meningococcal disease is at an historic low (0.18 per 100,000), with fewer than 600 cases reported annually during 2012 to 2014 (www. cdc.gov/mmwr). Until the early 2000s meningococcal disease incidence had a cyclical pattern, with peaks in incidence every 7 to 10 years and average incidence at 1.0 per 100,000 (**Fig. 3**). Since that time, the incidence has declined for 4 serogroups (B, C, W, and Y). Coverage among adolescents with at least 1 dose of MenACWY is high, but incidence has also declined for serogroup B, for which vaccines have been only recently licensed. Although meningococcal outbreaks comprise only 2% of the annual meningococcal cases in the United States, the onset, magnitude, and duration of these outbreaks is unpredictable, making outbreak control with vaccination challenging.[3,17]

For the last several years, the incidence of serogroup B meningococcal disease has remained stable and low in the United States, with the highest rates among infants younger than 12 months. There is currently no licensed serogroup B vaccine in the United States for children younger than 10 years. Among adolescents aged 11 through 23 years there are approximately 50 to 60 cases of serogroup B disease annually. However, as outbreaks of serogroup C have been reduced on college campuses with high uptake of MenACWY vaccine, several outbreaks of serogroup B meningococcal disease have occurred on college campuses since 2008.[18,19] Before licensure of the currently available MenB vaccines, 2 universities vaccinated, in response to

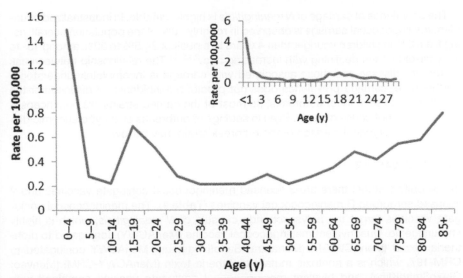

Fig. 2. Rate of meningococcal disease (per 100,000 population), by age: United States, 2002 to 2011. (*From* Cohn AC, MacNeil JR, Clark TA, et al. Prevention and control of meningococcal disease: recommendations of the Advisory Committee on Immunization Practices (ACIP). MMWR Recomm Rep 2013;62(RR–2):1–28.)

outbreaks on their campuses, with MenB-4C (Bexsero, Novartis Vaccines), which was approved by the Food and Drug Administration for investigational use to control these outbreaks.[19] Although outbreaks on college campuses have resulted in several cases, including deaths, the estimated overall incidence of serogroup B meningococcal disease on college campuses (0.09 per 100,000) is similar to or lower than the incidence in all persons aged 18 through 23 years (0.14 per 100,000) (CDC and Advisory Committee on Immunization Practices [ACIP], June 2015).

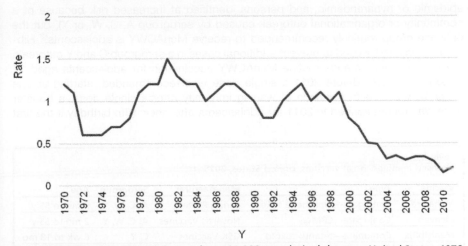

Fig. 3. Rate of meningococcal disease (per 100,000 population), by year: United States, 1970 to 2011. (*From* Cohn AC, MacNeil JR, Clark TA, et al. Prevention and control of meningococcal disease: recommendations of the Advisory Committee on Immunization Practices (ACIP). MMWR Recomm Rep 2013;62(RR–2):1–28.)

The prevalence of carriage of *N meningitidis* is highly variable. In industrialized countries, meningococcal carriage is observed in roughly 10% of the population overall, rising from 2% in children younger than 4 years to a peak of 24.5% to 32% among 15- to 24-year-olds, then declining with increasing age.[2,20,21] The relationship between risk factors for disease and those associated with carriage is incompletely understood. Furthermore, carriage prevalence does not predict the incidence of disease nor the occurrence or severity of outbreaks, as most of the carried strains are nonencapsulated and do not cause disease. Even in settings of outbreaks or in hyperendemic disease, nasopharyngeal carriage of the outbreak strain may be low.[22]

AVAILABLE VACCINES

In the United States there are 3 licensed meningococcal conjugate vaccines and 2 licensed serogroup B meningococcal vaccines (**Table 1**). The meningococcal conjugate vaccines target the polysaccharide capsule of *N meningitidis*, which is highly immunogenic. Quadrivalent meningococcal vaccine (MenACWY) conjugated to diphtheria toxoid (MenACWY-D) (Menactra; Sanofi Pasteur), MenACWY conjugated to CRM-197, which is a nontoxic mutant diphtheria toxin (MenACWY-CRM) (Menveo; GlaxoSmithKline), and bivalent meningococcal conjugate vaccine combined with *Haemophilus influenzae* type b (Hib) vaccine conjugated to tetanus toxoid (Hib-MenCY-TT) (MenHibrix; GlaxoSmithKline), all protect against serogroups C and Y, which cause approximately two-thirds of cases in the United States. MenACWY vaccines also protect against serogroups A and W, which allows them to also be used as travel vaccines for persons traveling to the Meningitis Belt during the dry season. These vaccines differ in their age indications: MenACWY-D is licensed for persons aged 9 months through 55 years, MenACWY-CRM is licensed for those aged 2 months through 55 years, and HibMenCY is licensed for children aged 2 through 18 months. These vaccines are all recommended for use in persons at increased risk for meningococcal disease (persons with persistent complement component deficiencies, persons with functional or anatomic asplenia, microbiologists routinely exposed to isolates of *N meningitidis*, travelers to an area where meningococcal disease is epidemic or hyperendemic, and persons identified at increased risk because of a community or organizational outbreak caused by serogroup A, C, W, or Y), but the only age group routinely recommended to receive MenACWY is adolescents.[3] Hib-Mency can only be used to prevent additional cases in a serogroup C and Y outbreak.

The ACIP recommends routine MenACWY vaccination for adolescents aged 11 through 18 years. Before 2011 a single dose was recommended, starting at age 11 or 12 years. With evidence of waning immunity after a single dose, a booster dose was recommended in 2011 for adolescents after their 16th birthday if the first

Table 1
Licensed meningococcal vaccines, United States, 2015

Vaccine	Type	Manufacturer	Serogroup	Age
Menactra	Conjugate—diphtheria toxoid	Sanofi Pasteur	A, C, W, Y	9 mo to 55 y
Menveo	Conjugate—CRM$_{197}$	Novartis Vaccines	A, C, W, Y	2 mo to 55 y
MenHibRix	Conjugate—tetanus toxoid	GSK Vaccines	C, Y	6 wk to 18 mo
Menomune	Polysaccharide	Sanofi Pasteur	A, C, W, Y	$\geq$2 y
Trumenba	Protein	Pfizer Vaccines	B	10–25 y
Bexsero	Protein	Novartis Vaccines	B	10–25 y

dose was received before age 16.[3] This booster dose was recommended to provide protection through late adolescence, when disease risk is increased. MenACWY coverage among teens aged 13 through 17 years in the United States was 79.3% in 2014 with at least 1 dose of MenACWY, and 28.5% for 2 doses.[23]

As the capsular polysaccharide antigen of serogroup B is similar to a human antigen, it is poorly immunogenic and not an appropriate target vaccine antigen. Therefore, noncapsular serogroup B vaccines were developed using innovative technology to identify immunogenic proteins that were (1) expressed on the outer surfaces of the organism in vivo and (2) produced a bactericidal immune response broadly, as there is more phenotypic variability in these proteins than in the polysaccharide capsule.[24,25] Two MenB vaccines were licensed in the United States for persons 10 through 25 years of age, and have the potential to prevent a substantial proportion of serogroup B disease.[26,27] However, because these vaccines are protein based, experience with these types of vaccines is limited.

MenB-4C consists of 3 recombinant proteins (neisserial adhesin A [NadA], factor H binding protein [FHbp] fusion protein, and neisserial heparin binding antigen [NHBA] fusion protein), and outer membrane vesicles containing outer membrane protein PorA serosubtype P1.4. MenB-4C is licensed as a 2-dose series, with doses administered at least 1 month apart, although in some studies MenB-4C doses were administered up to 6 months apart. MenB-FHbp consists of 2 purified recombinant FHbp antigens. One antigen from each FHbp subfamily (A and B) is included in the vaccine. MenB-FHbp is licensed as a 3-dose series, with the second and third doses administered 2 and 6 months after the first dose. Both of these vaccines were licensed in the United States under an accelerated approval process, and additional safety and efficacy data are needed to better understand which proportion of strains causing serogroup B meningococcal disease will be prevented, the impact of these vaccines on nasopharyngeal carriage, and whether additional booster doses are needed for longer-term protection.

The ACIP recommends MenB vaccines routinely for persons 10 years of age or older who are at increased risk for meningococcal disease (persons with persistent complement component deficiencies, persons with functional or anatomic asplenia, microbiologists routinely exposed to isolates of N meningitidis, persons identified at increased risk because of a community or organizational outbreak).[5] Recommendations for use of MenB vaccines in adolescents are not yet available.

Globally, devastating epidemics of serogroup A meningococcal disease occurred in the Meningitis Belt of sub-Saharan Africa.[28] A MenA tetanus toxoid conjugate vaccine, called MenAfriVac (PsA-TT), was developed by a collaborative partnership, the Meningitis Vaccine Project, and is available for approximately 40 US cents per dose.[29] In 2010, PsA-TT was licensed in 1- to 29-year-olds and in 2011 was prequalified by the World Health Organization for use in Africa. Since September 2010, more than 200 million people have been vaccinated throughout the Meningitis Belt. As the first phase of mass vaccination is completed in the region, countries are developing plans to introduce the vaccine either through the routine infant immunization program or through periodic catch-up campaigns for young children (www.meningvax.org).

IMPACT OF VACCINATION ON DISEASE CONTROL

As the current United States adolescent MenACWY program has become more established, the first impact of the program on rates of serogroups C, Y, and W meningococcal disease have been observed. The incidence of serogroups C, Y, and W has decreased by 80% between 2004/2005 and 2012/2013 among 11- to 19-year-olds.

A similar decline in incidence has not been observed among age groups not routinely receiving conjugate vaccines, including infants younger than 1 year and persons aged 20 years and older[3] (CDC, unpublished data, 2015). Estimates from a large case-control study evaluating 1 of the 2 MenACWY vaccines, MenACWY-D, in the United States suggest high vaccine effectiveness early after vaccination, but 2 to 5 years after vaccination vaccine effectiveness wanes to 50% to 60%.[3] The booster dose recommendation was made to ensure that antibody levels remained high through late adolescence, when disease risk increases.

The impact of PsA-TT vaccine in Africa has been extraordinary. Burkina Faso, the first country to vaccinate nationwide, achieved more than 94% coverage during campaigns in late 2010. In the first year after PsA-TT vaccination in Burkina Faso, the incidence of meningitis fell by 99.8% and there were no cases of serogroup A meningococcal disease among vaccinated persons.[11] Furthermore, 1 year after the PsA-TT campaign there were no carriers of serogroup A N meningitidis in more than 5000 persons sampled.[30] These results have been replicated in other countries, and serogroup A epidemics have virtually been eliminated in the region.[31]

CHALLENGES AND OPPORTUNITIES

In 2015, for the first time there are vaccines available that protect against the 4 serogroups that cause the most meningococcal illness the United States. At present, these vaccines are not licensed or used routinely in all age groups, and do not provide life-long protection for a disease that occurs in all age groups. Serogroup C and Y meningococcal outbreaks have virtually been eliminated on college campuses, although there have been outbreaks among other age groups. Even with high MenACWY vaccine coverage in adolescents and historically low disease incidence in all age groups, cases and outbreaks of meningococcal disease will continue to occur. Health care providers and public health providers need to maintain vigilance to recognize cases and outbreaks of meningococcal disease early.

Much remains to be understood regarding the long-term safety, duration of protection, and impact of carriage of MenB vaccines. Although the bactericidal response to these protein antigens is not as strong as the bactericidal response to the polysaccharide (and require multiple doses), these antigens are expressed on all serogroups and therefore may protect more broadly against N meningitidis. The multi-dose series may be challenging to implement, especially in adolescents. However, integrating MenB vaccines into the adolescent immunization program may provide the opportunity for additional visits to complete the human papillomavirus 3-dose series, receive the booster MenACWY dose, or for adolescents to receive the annual influenza vaccine.

With the enormous impact of PsA-TT vaccine on the Meningitis Belt comes the challenge of ensuring continued protection in new birth cohorts, and maintaining a strong infrastructure for disease detection and monitoring. Recently, serogroups W, X, and, in 2014 and 2015 serogroup C, have caused focal outbreaks in the region.[13,32] This fact highlights the need for multivalent conjugate vaccines in the region, and the challenges of eradicating meningococcal outbreaks completely.

RESEARCH NEEDS

Although the incidence of meningococcal disease has remained low for more than 10 years, the reasons for the change in epidemiology are unknown. Therefore, high-quality disease surveillance remains important to detect potential changes in epidemiology that might affect vaccine policy decisions. In addition, continued monitoring of disease-causing strains of N meningitidis can identify changes in the organism that may affect vaccine effectiveness, especially for serogroup B.

Additional studies for newly licensed MenB vaccines are critical, including the need to assess the breadth of strain coverage and monitor vaccine safety. These vaccines were licensed using immunologic correlates of protection, similarly to licensure of conjugate vaccines, but the limited data available on antibody persistence suggest rapid waning of antibodies after vaccination, and continued studies on duration of protection are needed. In addition, the potential impact of MenB vaccines on carriage and herd immunity is unknown, as is the potential impact of selection pressure on circulating strains from vaccine introduction.

Finally, developing affordable multivalent conjugate meningococcal vaccines for sub-Saharan Africa will have the greatest global health impact. Meningococcal vaccines have pushed vaccine innovation in new directions, both technologically, through the development of serogroup B vaccines, and functionally, through the collaboration to develop an affordable vaccine to be made available to a region of the world with limited resources. Although the epidemiology of meningococcal disease is never predictable, the high cost of the disease on persons, families, and communities makes the prevention of meningococcal disease a constant high priority globally and in the United States.

REFERENCES

1. Cohn AC, MacNeil JR, Harrison LH, et al. Changes in Neisseria meningitidis disease epidemiology in the United States, 1998-2007: implications for prevention of meningococcal disease. Clin Infect Dis 2010;50(2):184–91.
2. Christensen H, May M, Bowen L, et al. Meningococcal carriage by age: a systematic review and meta-analysis. Lancet Infect Dis 2010;10(12):853–61.
3. Cohn AC, MacNeil JR, Clark TA, et al. Prevention and control of meningococcal disease: recommendations of the Advisory Committee on Immunization Practices (ACIP). MMWR Recomm Rep 2013;62(RR–2):1–28.
4. Bilukha OO, Rosenstein N. Prevention and control of meningococcal disease. Recommendations of the Advisory Committee on Immunization Practices (ACIP). MMWR Recomm Rep 2005;54(RR–7):1–21.
5. Folaranmi T, Rubin L, Martin SW, et al. Use of serogroup B meningococcal vaccines in persons aged >/=10 years at increased risk for serogroup B meningococcal disease: recommendations of the Advisory Committee on Immunization Practices, 2015. MMWR Morb Mortal Wkly Rep 2015;64(22):608–12.
6. Harrison LH, Shutt KA, Schmink SE, et al. Population structure and capsular switching of invasive Neisseria meningitidis isolates in the pre-meningococcal conjugate vaccine era—United States, 2000-2005. J Infect Dis 2010;201(8): 1208–24.
7. Mayer LW, Reeves MW, Al-Hamdan N, et al. Outbreak of W135 meningococcal disease in 2000: not emergence of a new W135 strain but clonal expansion within the electophoretic type-37 complex. J Infect Dis 2002;185(11):1596–605.
8. Ladhani SN, Lucidarme J, Newbold LS, et al. Invasive meningococcal capsular group Y disease, England and Wales, 2007-2009. Emerg Infect Dis 2012;18(1): 63–70.
9. Campbell H, Saliba V, Borrow R, et al. Targeted vaccination of teenagers following continued rapid endemic expansion of a single meningococcal group W clone (sequence type 11 clonal complex), United Kingdom 2015. Euro Surveill 2015;20(28):1–5.

10. Trotter CL, Andrews NJ, Kaczmarski EB, et al. Effectiveness of meningococcal serogroup C conjugate vaccine 4 years after introduction. Lancet 2004;364(9431): 365–7.

11. Novak RT, Kambou JL, Diomande FV, et al. Serogroup A meningococcal conjugate vaccination in Burkina Faso: analysis of national surveillance data. Lancet Infect Dis 2012;12(10):757–64.

12. Daugla DM, Gami JP, Gamougam K, et al. Effect of a serogroup A meningococcal conjugate vaccine (PsA-TT) on serogroup A meningococcal meningitis and carriage in Chad: a community study [corrected]. Lancet 2014;383(9911):40–7.

13. Funk A, Uadiale K, Kamau C, et al. Sequential outbreaks due to a new strain of Neisseria meningitidis serogroup C in northern Nigeria, 2013-14. PLoS Curr 2014;6. Available at: http://www.ncbi.nlm.nih.gov/pmc/articles/PMC4322033/.

14. Rosenstein NE, Perkins BA, Stephens DS, et al. Meningococcal disease. N Engl J Med 2001;344(18):1378–88.

15. Wu HM, Harcourt BH, Hatcher CP, et al. Emergence of ciprofloxacin-resistant Neisseria meningitidis in North America. N Engl J Med 2009;360(9):886–92.

16. Harrison LH, Trotter CL, Ramsay ME. Global epidemiology of meningococcal disease. Vaccine 2009;27(Suppl 2):B51–63.

17. Jackson LA, Schuchat A, Reeves MW, et al. Serogroup C meningococcal outbreaks in the United States. An emerging threat. JAMA 1995;273(5):383–9.

18. Mandal S, Wu HM, MacNeil JR, et al. Prolonged university outbreak of meningococcal disease associated with a serogroup B strain rarely seen in the United States. Clin Infect Dis 2013;57(3):344–8.

19. McNamara LA, Shumate AM, Johnsen P, et al. First use of a serogroup B meningococcal vaccine in the US in response to a university outbreak. Pediatrics 2015; 135(5):798–804.

20. Trotter CL, Gay NJ, Edmunds WJ. The natural history of meningococcal carriage and disease. Epidemiol Infect 2006;134(3):556–66.

21. Caugant DA, Hoiby EA, Magnus P, et al. Asymptomatic carriage of Neisseria meningitidis in a randomly sampled population. J Clin Microbiol 1994;32(2): 323–30.

22. Kristiansen PA, Diomande F, Wei SC, et al. Baseline meningococcal carriage in Burkina Faso before the introduction of a meningococcal serogroup A conjugate vaccine. Clin Vaccine Immunol 2011;18(3):435–43.

23. Reagan-Steiner S, Yankey D, Jeyarajah J, et al. National, Regional, State, and Selected Local Area Vaccination Coverage Among Adolescents Aged 13-17 Years - United States, 2014. MMWR 2015;64(29):784–92.

24. Sette A, Rappuoli R. Reverse vaccinology: developing vaccines in the era of genomics. Immunity 2010;33(4):530–41.

25. Giuliani MM, Adu-Bobie J, Comanducci M, et al. A universal vaccine for serogroup B meningococcus. Proc Natl Acad Sci U S A 2006;103(29):10834–9.

26. MenB-4C, Bexsero [package insert]. Available at: http://www.fda.gov/downloads/BiologicsBloodVaccines/Vaccines/ApprovedProducts/UCM431447.pdf. Accessed September 28, 2015.

27. MenB-FHbp, Trumenba [package insert]. Available at: http://www.fda.gov/downloads/BiologicsBloodVaccines/Vaccines/ApprovedProducts/UCM421139.pdf. Accessed September 28, 2015.

28. LaForce M, Ravenscroft N, Mamoudou D, et al. Epidemic meningitis due to Group A Neisseria meningitidis in the African meningitis belt: a persistent problem with an imminent solution. Vaccine 2009;27(Suppl 2):B13–9.

29. LaForce FM, Okwo-Bele JM. Eliminating epidemic Group A meningococcal men-ingitis in Africa through a new vaccine. Health Aff (Millwood) 2011;30(6):1049–57.
30. Kristiansen PA, Ba AK, Ouedraogo AS, et al. Persistent low carriage of serogroup A *Neisseria meningitidis* two years after mass vaccination with the meningococcal conjugate vaccine, MenAfriVac. BMC Infect Dis 2014;14:663.
31. Gamougam K, Daugla DM, Toralta J, et al. Continuing effectiveness of serogroup A meningococcal conjugate vaccine, Chad, 2013. Emerg Infect Dis 2015;21(1): 115–8.
32. Delrieu I, Yaro S, Tamekloe TAS, et al. Emergence of epidemic *Neisseria meningitidis* serogroup X meningitis in Togo and Burkina Faso. PLoS One 2011;6(5):e19513.

Pneumococcal Disease in the Era of Pneumococcal Conjugate Vaccine

Inci Yildirim, MD, MSc[a,b,c], Kimberly M. Shea, PhD, MPH[b], Stephen I. Pelton, MD[a,b,c],*

KEYWORDS

- Pneumococcal disease • Pneumococcal conjugate vaccine
- Invasive pneumococcal disease • Pneumococcal meningitis
- Pneumococcal pneumonia

KEY POINTS

- Universal immunization of infants and toddlers with pneumococcal conjugate vaccines has resulted in decreases in invasive pneumococcal disease, all-cause pneumonia, empyema, mastoiditis, acute otitis media, and complicated otitis media.
- The impact of pneumococcal conjugate vaccine extends beyond those immunized to children too young to be immunized, children unable to respond to the vaccine, and adults in the community as a result of herd effect.
- Children with comorbid conditions have higher rates of pneumococcal disease and increased case fatality rates compared with otherwise healthy children.
- Treatment of pneumococcal disease requires an approach that considers site of infection, antimicrobial susceptibility patterns in the community, and severity of illness.

The universal immunization of infants and toddlers with pneumococcal conjugate vaccine (PCV) in the United States beginning in 2000 heralded a new era for pneumococcal disease prevention. Conjugate vaccines were immunogenic in young infants, prevented vaccine type invasive pneumococcal disease (IPD), pneumonia and otitis

Disclosure Statement: Dr S.I. Pelton receives IIR research funding (through BUMC) from Pfizer (Grant no WS951925) and Merck Vaccines (Grant no 303202) and Honorarium or consulting fees from Pfizer for activities related to pneumococcal conjugate vaccine/pneumococcal disease. Dr K.M. Shea receives IIR research funding (through BUMC) from Pfizer and consulting fees from Pfizer for activities related to pneumococcal diseases.
[a] Section of Pediatric Infectious Diseases, Department of Pediatrics, Boston University Medical Center, Boston, MA 02118, USA; [b] Department of Epidemiology, Boston University School of Public Health, 715 Albany Street, Boston, MA 02118, USA; [c] Maxwell Finland Laboratory for Infectious Diseases, 670 Albany Street, Boston, MA 02118, USA
* Corresponding author. Department of Epidemiology, Boston University School of Public Health, Room 322, 715 Albany Street, Boston, MA 02118.
E-mail address: spelton@bu.edu

Infect Dis Clin N Am 29 (2015) 679–697
http://dx.doi.org/10.1016/j.idc.2015.07.009

id.theclinics.com

media, and decreased nasopharyngeal colonization with vaccine serotypes leading to a herd effect that affected all age groups. However, new challenges emerged that would eventually lead to second-generation conjugates that included a larger number of serotypes to address both replacement disease (increases in disease owing to non-vaccine serotypes) and providing more expansive coverage for the global community. Postlicensure studies provided new insights into the importance of serotype distribution among carriage isolates and how the event-to-carrier ratio for a specific serotype permits us to understand the substantial decline in IPD in the absence of a decline in overall pneumococcal colonization. The limitation of current diagnostic tools for pneumococcal pneumonia became apparent from the discord between the prevalence of diagnosed pneumococcal pneumonia in studies of pediatric pneumonia compared with the observed decline in all-cause pneumonia associated with pneumococcal vaccine uptake in the community.[1,2] Despite the progress in prevention, pneumococcal disease continues to disproportionately impact children in low-income countries and those with comorbid conditions (in high-income countries) and remains a major cause of mortality and morbidity.

EPIDEMIOLOGY

Nasopharyngeal colonization with Streptococcus pneumoniae is an initial step in the pathogenesis of pneumococcal disease. Asymptomatic carriage is common with reported prevalence ranging from 11% to 93%; carriage varies with age, environment, the presence of upper respiratory infections, and population studied.[3,4] Risk factors for pneumococcal carriage include age younger than 2 years, exposure to overcrowding and household smoking, attendance at out-of-home child care, winter season, and lack of breast feeding.[5] Initial acquisition of pneumococci occurs earlier in low-income countries, (as early as the first month of life) compared with high-income countries and peaks at 2 to 3 years of age.[4,6] Among school-age children, 20% to 60% may be colonized, whereas only 5% to 10% of adults are colonized. The duration of carriage also varies and is generally longer in children than in adults.[6] The relationship of carriage to the development of natural immunity is poorly understood, but the prevalence of nasopharyngeal carriage declines over time, suggesting that colonization elicits protection.[7] The impact of conjugated vaccines on pneumococcal carriage has been dramatic; vaccination has resulted in near elimination of vaccine serotypes and increased prevalence of nonvaccine serotypes, with little change in the overall rate of pneumococcal colonization. Changing serotype distributions in the nasopharynx has led to a subsequent reduction in IPD, as most nonvaccine serotypes have a lower likelihood of causing disease once colonization has been established, and decreased transmission of vaccine serotypes to under- or unimmunized children and adults, also resulting in lower rates of IPD in under- or unimmunized children and adults.[8]

Most S pneumoniae serotypes are found to cause serious disease, but of the 92 known pneumococcal serotypes, 10 serotypes account for nearly 62% of invasive disease worldwide.[9] The rank order and serotype prevalence differ over time, by age group and by geographic area. In the United States, before widespread use of 7-valent pneumococcal conjugate vaccine (PCV7), serotypes 4, 6B, 9V, 18C, 19F, and 23F were the most common serotypes isolated from blood or cerebrospinal fluid (CSF) and were responsible for 80% of the invasive infections in children younger than 5 years.[10] Serotypes 6B, 9V, 19F, and 23F also accounted for approximately 80% of penicillin-nonsusceptible isolates. Pneumococcal disease is mostly episodic; however, pneumococci are transmitted from person to person by respiratory droplets, and outbreaks have occurred in overcrowded enclosed settings such as military barracks, homeless shelters, prisons, and childcare facilities most often caused by serotype 1, 5, or 8.[5,11]

The age distribution of IPD has changed with the universal immunization of infants and toddlers with conjugate vaccine. Before 2000, IPD was seen most often in children younger than 5 years and had a second peak after age 65.[12] Currently, the highest rates of IPD are seen in persons older than 65 years with a smaller peak in children younger than 5 (**Fig. 1**) and an increasing proportion of pediatric cases in the 5- to 18-year age group.[7,12,13] Type-specific antibodies are passively transferred from the mother and are protective for the first months of life in full-term infants. The peak incidence of IPD in children occurs between 6 and 11 months of age as maternal antibody declines.[14] In neonatal pneumococcal infections, the organism is usually acquired from the maternal genital tract, and both early-onset and late-onset disease has been identified. Bacteremia without a known site of infection is the most common presentation of IPD among children 2 years of age and younger, accounting for approximately 70% of invasive disease in this age group, whereas bacteremic pneumonia accounts 12% to 16% of cases.[7] Before routine use of pneumococcal conjugate vaccine, meningitis was most commonly seen in children between age 6 to 18 months with an approximate rate of 10 cases per 100,000 population and an 8% case-fatality rate among children in the United States.[15] Most cases of pneumococcal bone and joint infections are in children 3 to 34 months old, whereas most pneumococcal pneumonia cases are seen in children between 3 and 60 months of age.[7] Pneumococci are also a common cause of acute otitis media and are detected in 28% to 55% of middle ear aspirates. The peak incidence of cause of acute otitis media in otherwise healthy children is between 6 and 18 months,

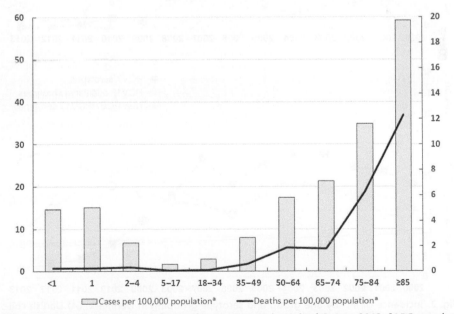

Fig. 1. Rates of pneumococcal disease by age groups in United States, 2013. [a]ABC population areas. (*From* Centers for Disease control and prevention. Active Bacterial core Surveillance (ABCs)/Emerging Infections Programs network (EIP). 2013. Available at: http://www.cdc.gov/abcs/reports-findings/survreports/spneu13.html. Accessed July 27, 2015.)

and, by age 12 months, more than 60% of children have had at least one episode of acute otitis media.

The impact of widespread PCV immunization of children on IPD has been substantial in all age groups. **Fig. 2** shows the decline in PCV7 serotypes after introduction of PCV7 in Denmark, the increase and subsequent decline in 13-valent conjugate vaccine (PCV13) serotypes after use of PCV7 and subsequent switch to PCV13, and the increase in disease attributable to nonvaccine serotypes.[16] In the United States, results from the Active Bacterial Core Surveillance Program conducted by the Centers for Disease Control and Prevention indicated that rate of IPD, in all age groups combined, decreased from an average of 24.3 cases per 100,000 persons in the

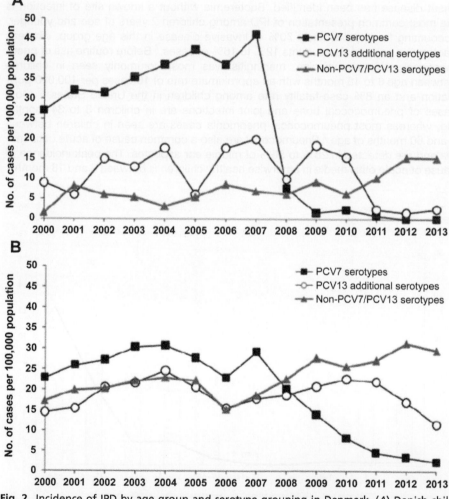

Fig. 2. Incidence of IPD by age group and serotype grouping in Denmark. (*A*) Danish children less than 2 years of age. (*B*) Danish adults ≥65 years of age. PCV7 was introduced in 2007 and PCV13 in 2010. (*From* Harboe ZB, Dalby T, Weinberger DM, et al. Impact of 13-valent pneumococcal conjugate vaccination in invasive pneumococcal disease incidence and mortality. Clin Infect Dis 2014;59:1069; with permission.)

prevaccine years (1998 and 1999) to 17.3 cases per 100,000 persons after the vaccine's introduction in 2001.[17] Invasive disease caused by vaccine serotypes declined more than 99% in children younger than 5 years, resulting in a 75% decline in overall IPD in this age group, which resulted from direct effects in vaccine recipients and the herd effect in unvaccinated children.[17,18] Because serotypes included in PCV7 accounted for most antibiotic-resistant strains, the proportion of resistant isolates also declined initially. The rate of disease caused by penicillin-nonsusceptible isolates decreased by 35% compared with that in the prevaccine year 1999 (6.3 cases per 100,000 individuals to 4.1 cases per 100,000 individuals).[17] After almost a decade of PCV7 use, some studies report an increasing incidence of IPD primarily caused by non-PCV7 serotypes (replacement disease). Singleton and colleagues[19] reported that replacement disease resulted in an incidence of IPD among native Alaskan children that exceed the incidence in the pre-PCV7 era. Yildirim and colleagues[13] identified that despite a sustained decrease in the overall incidence of IPD in Massachusetts, disease caused by non-PCV7 serotypes such as 19A, 7F, and 15B/C increased and caused most IPD in children from 2007 to 2009 (**Fig. 3**). Emerging nonvaccine serotypes, mostly 1, 7F, 12F, 19A, 22F, and 24F were associated with an increase in IPD rates among children in Europe.[20,21] The increase in disease caused by nonvaccine serotypes was not limited to IPD; pneumococcal empyema increased in both the United States and Europe,[22–24] an increase in cases of mastoiditis and unresponsive otitis media caused by serotype 19A was observed,[25] and increasing cases of pneumococcal hemolytic uremic syndrome[26,27] were reported.

The erosion of PCV7 effectiveness for IPD from an increase in disease caused by nonvaccine serotypes and the increasing concern about increasing case numbers of empyema, mastoiditis, and unresponsive otitis media led to the introduction of a

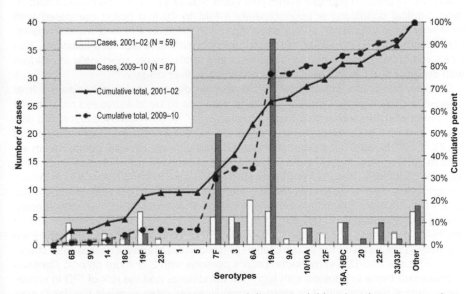

Fig. 3. Serotypes causing invasive pneumococcal disease in children less than 18 years of age in Massachusetts. Comparison of 2001 to 2002 and 2009 to 2010. (*From* Yildirim I, Stevenson A, Hsu KK, et al. Evolving picture of invasive pneumococcal disease in Massachusetts children: a comparison of disease in 2007–2009 with earlier periods. Pediatr Infect Dis J 2012;31(10):1019; with permission.)

second-generation, 13-valent conjugate vaccine (PCV13) targeting 6 additional sero-types in 2010 (1, 3, 5, 6A, 7F, 19A). Within 6 months after introduction of PCV13, a rapid reduction in PCV13 type IPD was observed in children younger than 5 years who were targeted for vaccination. Moore and colleagues[28] reported that compared with what would have been predicted in the absence of PCV13, overall incidence of IPD in June 2013, was 64% lower, whereas incidence of disease caused by the unique PCV13 serotypes declined 93%. A similar reduction, through herd protection, was observed among adults. In all age groups, changes in incidence were driven princi-pally by declines in IPD caused by serotypes 19A and 7F.

PNEUMOCOCCAL DISEASE IN CHILDREN WITH COMORBID CONDITIONS

Several recent studies found that although pneumococcal vaccination has substan-tially reduced IPD incidence in all risk groups, persons with immunodeficiency or chronic medical conditions continue to suffer a disproportionate burden of pneumo-coccal disease.[29–32]

For example, in human immunodeficiency virus (HIV)-infected adults, the incidence of PCV7-type IPD decreased by 88% after the introduction of PCV7 in children as a result of herd (indirect) effects, but the rate of PCV7-type IPD in this population per-sists at 40-fold higher than the rate among healthy adults in the same age group.[33] IPD risk is highest among children and adults with immunocompromised immune sys-tems caused by congenital or acquired immunodeficiency, immunosuppressive ther-apy, functional (eg, sickle cell disease) or anatomic asplenia, chronic renal failure, or nephrotic syndrome.[7,32,34] In immunocompromised adults 18 to 64 years of age, the incidence of IPD is 100 to 400 cases per 100,000[30,33] compared with approximately 9 cases per 1000,000 in otherwise healthy adults in that age group.[31] Similarly, the risk of IPD in children younger than 5 years and 5 to 17 years with immunocomprom-ising medical conditions is approximately 4-fold to 40-fold higher compared with otherwise healthy children of the same age.[29] In addition to being more frequent, the outcome of IPD in children with comorbid conditions is also less favorable. Van Hoek and colleagues[35] reported increased case fatality rates, specifically in children with asplenia and chronic cardiac, pulmonary, and liver disease.[32]

Children and adults with chronic cardiovascular disease, pulmonary disease, liver disease, kidney disease, and CSF leakage continue to be at increased risk for IPD compared with persons without these conditions.[35–37] More recently, asthma and dia-betes have also been identified as independent risk factors for IPD in children and adults.[29,30,38] Several large population-based studies were recently conducted in ef-forts to better characterize the magnitude of risk associated with individual underlying medical conditions. Results from these studies indicate that the risk of IPD in immu-nocompetent children who have one or more of the chronic medical conditions for which the Advisory Committee on Immunization Practices (ACIP) currently recom-mends pneumococcal vaccination,[35] is 2-fold to 4-fold higher[29] and risk of IPD in adults is 3-fold higher.[30] In addition, the risk of IPD in immunocompetent persons sub-stantially increases with the accumulation of concurrent chronic illnesses (risk stack-ing).[31] The risk of IPD in immunocompetent persons with 2 or more chronic illnesses approximate those in persons with high-risk conditions, and the risk of IPD in immu-nocompetent persons with 3 or more chronic illnesses often exceeds the risk in per-sons with high-risk conditions (**Fig. 4**).[29]

In part, the serotype distribution in children with comorbid conditions explains the persistence of increased risk. Several studies identified an increased proportion of IPD caused by nonvaccine serotypes in children with comorbid conditions.[32,39]

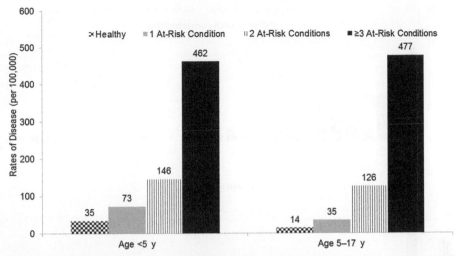

Fig. 4. Rates of pneumococcal pneumonia in children with at risk conditions compared with otherwise healthy children. (*Adapted from* Pelton SI, Weycker D, Farkouh RA, et al. Risk of pneumococcal disease in children with chronic medical conditions in the era of pneumococcal conjugate vaccine. Clin Infect Dis 2014;59:620; with permission.)

Ladhani and colleagues[40] reported that children with comorbid conditions have a broader spectrum of serotypes including those with a lower likelihood of causing disease after colonization (**Fig. 5**). These observations have important implications and provide support for the ACIP recommendations for immunization with 23-valent pneumococcal polysaccharide vaccine in children with specified at-risk conditions.[12]

LABORATORY DIAGNOSIS

Conventional practice for the diagnosis of pneumococcal disease continues to rely on the isolation of *S pneumoniae* in culture from blood or normally sterile body sites such as pleural fluid, CSF, synovial fluid, or cardiac vegetation. Pneumococcal isolation is jeopardized by prior antibiotic therapy; therefore, cultures should be obtained before antimicrobial treatment is started. The bacterium typically grows within 18 to 24 hours of inoculation of the culture media. In his historical study from early 20th century, Rosenow[41] found that 90% of patients with pneumococcal pneumonia had positive blood cultures. However rates of positive blood culture depend on the technique, volume of the sample, and other similar factors and can be only 3% to 8% among adults hospitalized with pneumonia, even lower in children. In more recent studies conducted before widespread use of pneumococcal vaccines, around 88% of the patients with pneumococcal meningitis were reported to have positive blood cultures.[42]

The most recent developments in laboratory diagnosis of pneumococcal infections have occurred with antigen detection assays. Rapid antigen tests such as latex agglutination or enzyme immunoassay tests targeting capsular polysaccharide have been used in testing sputum, CSF, and urine but were found to be poorly sensitive and not specific enough to be of clinical value, especially in children. An immunochromatographic urine antigen assay (Binax NOW *S pneumoniae* test; Binax Inc, Portland, ME) targeting the C polysaccharide cell wall antigen that is common to all strains of *S pneumoniae* was found to be promising for diagnosis of community-acquired pneumonia in adult patients, however, leads to high false-positive results. In one study, 51% of

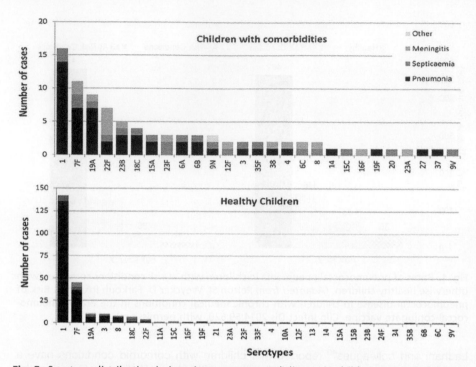

Fig. 5. Serotype distribution in invasive pneumococcal disease in children age 5 to 15 years with and without comorbidity. (*Adapted from* Ladhani SN, Andrews NJ, Waight P, et al. Invasive pneumococcal disease, comorbidities, and polysaccharide vaccine use in children aged 5-15 years in England and Wales. Clin Infect Dis 2014;58:521; with permission.)

healthy children tested positive[43] in the absence of any clinical manifestations of pneumonia or bacteremia, presumably because of nasopharyngeal colonization only. The same test when used on CSF samples was 100% sensitive for identification of S pneumoniae in pyogenic CSF with very high specificity compared with the nonpneumococcal cases.[44,45]

The role of nucleic acid amplification tests in diagnosis of pneumococcal infections has yet to be fully clarified. Polymerase chain reaction (PCR)-based techniques have the advantage of detecting both the viable and nonviable S pneumoniae in clinical samples and may be used alone or in combination with other tests for diagnosis of pneumococcal infections. PCR detects S pneumoniae in blood samples with a sensitivity ranging from 29% to 100% in children with pneumonia.[46] When applied to CSF samples, the sensitivity and specificity have been reported as 92% to 100%.[47] Quantitative PCR is also suggested as a tool to distinguish colonization from infection, with a higher bacterial burden among individuals with in invasive pneumococcal disease. However, the value of quantitation appears more promising in adults than in children.

Matrix-assisted laser desorption ionization time-of-flight mass spectrometry has been adapted for the routine identification of microorganisms in clinical microbiology laboratories in the last 10 years and theoretically has the potential to identify any organism from a positive blood culture.[48] Although this technology is reported to reduce the cost and time to result of bacterial identification,[49] blood culture samples require processing before matrix-assisted laser desorption ionization time-of-flight mass spectrometry analysis to remove nonbacterial proteins, such as serum proteins and hemoglobin, and it fails to reliably differentiate *S pneumoniae* from *Streptococcus mitis*.[50]

Other rapid molecular methods using real-time multiplexed nucleic acid amplification tests (eg, Film Array System; IdahoTechnology, Salt Lake City, UT)[51] are being developed to decrease the detection time and have been adopted for diagnosis of pneumococcal infections and infections caused by other bacteria (eg, *Staphylococcus aureus*). These approaches make up a potential point-of-care diagnostic tool with high sensitivity and specificity in direct identification of pneumococci, especially from positive blood culture bottles.[52] However further studies analyzing the clinical significance of positive results in samples from patients with pneumococcal infections are warranted.

However, despite developments in laboratory diagnostics, a microbiological diagnosis is still not made in most cases of IPD, particularly for pneumococcal pneumonia, largely as a result of the problems associated with obtaining high-quality lower respiratory tract samples for testing and with uncertainty regarding the differentiation of infection from colonization. The microscopic demonstration of numerous gram-positive diplococci in a sputum sample with less than 10 squamous epithelial cells and greater than 25 polymorphonuclear cells per low-power field (magnification, × 100) or ≥10 leukocytes for each squamous epithelial cell is strongly suggestive of pneumococcal pneumonia (**Fig. 6**).[53] Transthoracic needle aspiration of infected lung parenchyma has the potential to improve the diagnostic yield, especially in children who may not produce sputum; however, the procedure is not justified in many patients with uncomplicated pneumonia.[54] Taken together, there is no easy way to establish the diagnosis of nonbacteremic pneumococcal infections, and increased efforts should be directed toward development of more sensitive and specific new diagnostic tools to help clinicians diagnose especially pneumococcal pneumonia.

TREATMENT

Treatment of pneumococcal disease requires an approach that considers site of infection, antimicrobial susceptibility patterns in the community, and severity of illness.

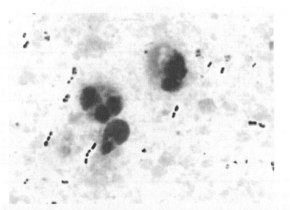

Fig. 6. Gram stain of a sputum sample showing *S pneumoniae* as gram-positive diplococci. (*From* Werno AM, Murdoch DR. Medical microbiology: laboratory diagnosis of invasive pneumococcal disease. Clin Infect Dis 2008;46:927; with permission.)

Pneumococcal Meningitis

Pneumococcal meningitis is associated with the greatest mortality and morbidity and requires effective therapy that will rapidly sterilize the central nervous system and limit the inflammatory response and its potential impact on cerebral blood perfusion, hypoxia, and cell death. Initial assessment must include evaluation of circulatory function and fluid status, as sepsis will frequently also be present. Attention to vital signs, mental status, urine output, and electrolyte management is critical for optimizing outcomes. Sufficient fluid should be provided to maintain normal systolic blood pressure, tissue perfusion, and urine output. Evaluation for inappropriate antidiuretic hormone secretion, manifest as hyponatremia, should be also included in the initial assessment.

In otherwise healthy children, initial antibiotic selection should include coverage for most common pathogens—S pneumoniae and Neisseria meningitidis in children older than 3 months and S pneumoniae, Group B streptococcus, Listeria monocytogenes, and enteric gram-negative bacteria in children younger than 3 months of age. Initial therapy should be administered intravenously to achieve adequate serum and CSF concentrations; intraosseous administration is appropriate, in unstable children, if venous access cannot be established. According to the 2004 Infectious Diseases Society of America practice guidelines for bacterial meningitis, vancomycin plus either ceftriaxone or cefotaxime is recommended for suspected bacterial meningitis.[55] We continue to use this combination despite the decline in serotype 19A prevalence in the community, as most recent data continues to identify cases of 19A disease in children.[32] As vancomycin penetrates the central nervous system (CNS) poorly, especially when administered with dexamethasone, higher dosing (70 mg/kg/d) is recommended initially (**Table 1**) specifically in children younger than 12 years.[56] Once the etiology is established and susceptibility determined, cefotaxime or ceftriaxone alone is adequate when susceptible pneumococci are causative. When the minimal inhibitory concentration (MIC) for cefotaxime is increased (MIC $\geq$0.5 µg/mL; considered intermediate resistance), a higher dose of cefotaxime (300 mg/kg/d) in combination with vancomycin (70 mg/kg/d) may achieve more rapid sterilization of the CSF (**Table 2**).[57] Although now less common since the introduction of PCV13, if high-level resistance to cefotaxime or ceftriaxone is present (MIC $\geq$2 µg/mL), rifampin added to the regimen enhances

Table 1				
Antibiotic dosing appropriate for pneumococcal meningitis				
	Total Daily Dose (Number of Doses per Day)		**Susceptible**
Antimicrobial Agent	**Adolescents**	**Infants and Children**	**Breakpoint (µg/mL)[a]**
Parenteral agents			
Penicillin G	24 million Units	300,000–400,000 units/kg	$\leq$0.06
Ampicillin	12 g	300 mg/kg	Penicillin $\leq$0.06
Ceftriaxone	4 g	100 mg/kg	$\leq$0.5
Cefotaxime	8–12 g	225–300 mg/kg	$\leq$0.5
Rifampin	600 mg	20 mg/kg	$\leq$0.5
Meropenem	6 g	120 mg/kg	$\leq$0.25
Vancomycin[b]	30–45 mg/kg	70–80 mg/kg	—

[a] Susceptibility breakpoint for agent shown unless specified otherwise.
[b] Dosing should be adjusted to achieve trough concentrations of 15 to 20 µg/mL for CNS infection.
    Adapted from Pelton SI, Jacobs MR. Pneumococcal infections. In: Cherry JD, Harrison GJ, Kaplan SL, editors. Feigin and Cherry's textbook of pediatric infectious diseases. 7th edition. Philadelphia: Elsevier Saunders; 2014. p. 1217; with permission.

Table 2
Specific recommendations for antimicrobial selection in pneumococcal meningitis based on penicillin and ceftriaxone susceptibility

Susceptibility	Standard Therapy	Alternative Therapies
Penicillin MIC		
<0.1 µg/mL	Penicillin G or ampicillin	Third-generation cephalosporin,[a] chloramphenicol
0.1–1.0 µg/mL[b]	Third-generation cephalosporin[a]	Cefepime, meropenem
2.0 µg/mL	Vancomycin plus a third-generation cephalosporin[c]	Fluoroquinolone[d]
Cefotaxime or ceftriaxone MIC		
1.0 µg/mL	Vancomycin plus a third-generation cephalosporin[c]	Fluoroquinolone[d]

[a] Ceftriaxone or cefotaxime.
[b] Ceftriaxone/cefotaxime-susceptible isolates.
[c] Consider addition of rifampin if the MIC of ceftriaxone is 12 mg/mL.
[d] Gatifloxacin or moxifloxacin.
  Adapted from Tunkel AR, Hartman BJ, Kaplan SL, et al. Practice guidelines for the management of bacterial meningitis. Clin Infect Dis 2004;39:1276.

the bactericidal activity in the CSF. Meropenem has been studied in children with bacterial meningitis and is found to have clinical and microbiologic outcomes similar to those of third-generation cephalosporins. Meropenem may also be effective in patients with pneumococcal meningitis caused by highly penicillin- and cephalosporin-resistant strains when the isolate is meropenem susceptible. Repeat lumbar puncture to evaluate sterilization of the CNS is not routinely performed. Indications for repeat lumbar puncture would include a failure to improve after 48 to 72 hours of antimicrobial therapy or possibly in the setting in which dexamethasone has been administered and a highly resistant pneumococci was isolated from CSF, as the use of steroids potentially could cloud the assessment of clinical response.

Reducing inflammation in the CNS is also found to be of benefit in animal models, children with meningitis caused by Haemophilus influenza type B and adults with pneumococcal meningitis. However, controversy persists regarding its use in children with pneumococcal meningitis. Infectious Diseases Society of America guidelines recommend adjunctive dexamethasone in a dose of 0.15 mg/kg every 6 hours for 2 to 4 days, initiated 10 to 20 minutes before (or at least concomitant with) the first antimicrobial dose. In contrast, The American Academy of Pediatrics Committee on Infectious Diseases suggests that dexamethasone therapy be considered for infants and children older than 6 weeks with pneumococcal meningitis after weighing the potential risks and benefits.[58] Our current approach is based on a case-by-case analysis; however, more often than not we favor its use in children with suspected bacterial meningitis and mental status changes or neurologic deficits on presentation. Adverse events have been uncommonly associated with use of dexamethasone in bacterial meningitis; gastrointestinal bleeding is the most common and recently delayed cerebral thrombosis after initial good recovery from pneumococcal meningitis has been reported in adults.[59]

Pneumococcal Pneumonia

The treatment of pneumococcal pneumonia presents a different challenge than that of meningitis, as achieving sufficient drug concentration in the lung and alveolar fluid is less challenging that in the CNS. Beta-lactam antibiotics (eg, amoxicillin, ceftriaxone) achieve high levels in the respiratory tract such that pneumococci with minimal inhibitory concentration of less than 8 μg/mL for penicillin and less than 4 μg/mL for ceftriaxone can be successfully treated. For pneumococcal pneumonia without complications, including disease caused by penicillin- and ceftriaxone-resistant pneumococci, amoxicillin is the drug of choice if the organism's MIC is less than 8 μg/mL. For pneumococci with an MIC of 8 μg/mL or higher, ceftriaxone (if MIC is <4 μg/mL) is first choice. Recovery from pneumococcal pneumonia may be prolonged especially when empyema or necrotizing pneumonia is present. The presence of cavitation, pneumatocele, or empyema requires a different approach. Ceftriaxone and vancomycin, in combination, is currently the initial regimen of choice with modification based on results of cultures. Such cases may require chest tube drainage or video-assisted thoracic surgery. Nearly all patients recover completely; however, the course may be prolonged with fever lasting up to 3 weeks and prolonged hospitalization.[60]

During the last decade, increasing numbers of cases of pneumococcal-related hemolytic uremic syndrome have been reported, most often associated with pneumonia and empyema.[26,27] The cases seem to occur in mostly infants and toddlers, often are caused by serotype 19A (but not exclusively) and are likely to progress to severe renal and hematologic disease often requiring dialysis and platelet and packed red blood cell transfusions.[27]

PREVENTION

Pneumococcal vaccines, both polysaccharide and conjugate formulations, are recommended by the ACIP for prevention of pneumococcal disease. Currently available 23-valent polysaccharide vaccine (PPSV23; Pneumovax, Merck & Company, Inc [Kenilworth, NJ, USA]) was licensed in the United States in 1983 and contains purified polysaccharide antigen (25 μg of each per dose) of 23 serotypes (1, 2, 3, 4, 5, 6B, 7F, 8, 9N, 9V, 10A, 11A, 12F, 14, 15B, 17F, 18C, 19A, 19F, 20, 22F, 23F, and 33F) that accounted for 90% of the invasive pneumococcal disease at the time of licensure.[7] PPSV23 induces antibody response in approximately 80% of healthy adult vaccinees within 2 to 3 weeks of immunization, and elevated antibody levels persist for at least 5 years. This vaccine is found to be effective against invasive pneumococcal disease with efficacy between 56% and 86% in healthy adults.[61] However, capsular polysaccharides used in the vaccine are T-independent immunogens and induce limited antibody response in young children, specifically younger than 2 years, which is the age group with highest incidence of pneumococcal infections.[62] Additional major caveats in the pediatric age group are polysaccharide antigens do not induce immunologic memory and fail to prime for booster response with the subsequent exposure, serotype-specific antibody levels decline rapidly after the immunization within 3 to 5 years, immunization does not reduce nasopharyngeal colonization, and efficacy against mucosal surface infection such as nonbacteremic pneumonia and otitis media is limited. Despite these limitations, the use of PPSV23 is still recommended for US children with increased risk of invasive pneumococcal disease, such as those with sickle cell disease or HIV infection, after they complete their conjugated vaccine series (**Table 3**).[63]

To address the problem of decreased immunogenicity, polysaccharide antigens have been covalently linked to protein carriers to induce T helper cell response. In February 2000, a 7-valent pneumococcal polysaccharide-protein conjugate vaccine (PCV7; Prevnar, Wyeth, Collegeville, PA) was licensed in the United States and contained serotypes 4, 6B, 9V, 14, 18C, 19F, and 23F.[7] A prelicensure clinical efficacy trial of PCV7 found 97.4% efficacy against IPD caused by vaccine serotypes among fully

Table 3
Medical conditions or other indications for administration of PCV13ᵃ and indications for PPSV23ᵇ administration and revaccination for children age 6 to18 yearsᶜ

Risk Group	Underlying Medical Condition	PCV13 Recommended	PPSV23 Recommended	PPSV23 Revaccination 5 y
Immunocompetent persons	Chronic heart diseaseᵈ	—	✓	—
	Chronic lung diseaseᵉ	—	✓	—
	Diabetes mellitus	—	✓	—
	Cerebrospinal fluid leaks	✓	✓	—
	Cochlear implants	✓	✓	—
	Alcoholism	—	✓	—
	Chronic liver disease	—	✓	—
	Cigarette smoking	—	✓	—
Persons with functiona or anatomic asplenia	Sickle cell disease/other hemaglobinopathies	✓	✓	✓
	Congenital or acquired asplenia	✓	✓	✓
Immunocompromised persons	Congenital or acquired immunodeficienciesᶠ	✓	✓	✓
	HIV infection	✓	✓	✓
	Chronic renal failure	✓	✓	✓
	Nephrotic syndrome	✓	✓	✓
	Leukemia	✓	✓	✓
	Lymphoma	✓	✓	✓
	Hodgkin disease	✓	✓	✓
	Generalized malignancy	✓	✓	✓
	Iatrogenic immunosuppressionᵍ	✓	✓	✓
	Solid organ transplant	✓	✓	✓
	Multiple myeloma	✓	✓	✓

[a] 13-valent pneumococca conjugate vaccine.

[b] 23-valent pneumococca polysaccharide vaccine.

[c] Children aged 2 to 5 years with chronic conditions (eg, heart disease or diabetes), immunocompromising conditions (eg, HIV, functional or anatomic asplenia (including sickle cell disease), cerebrospinal fluid leaks, or cochlear implants, and who have not previously received PCV13, have been recommended to receive PCV13 since 2010.

[d] Including congestive heart failure and cardiomyopathies.

[e] Including chronic obstructive pulmonary disease, emphysema, and asthma.

[f] Includes B-(humoral) or T-lymphocyte deficiency, complement deficiency, complement deficiencies (particularly C1, C2, C3, and C4 deficiencies), and phagocytic disorders (excluding chronic granulomatous disease).

[g] Diseases requiring treatment with immunosuppressive drugs, including long-term systemic corticosteroids and radiation therapy.

From Centers for Disease Control and Prevention (CDC). Use of 13-valent pneumococcal conjugate vaccine and 23-valent pneumococcal polysaccharide vaccine among children aged 6-18 years with immunocompromising conditions: recommendations of the Advisory Committee on Immunization Practices (ACIP). MMWR Morb Mortal Wkly Rep 2013;62:521–4.

vaccinated infants.[64] The safety, efficacy, and effectiveness in practice of PCV7 and other pneumococcal conjugate vaccines have been established in multiple settings in both high-income and low-income countries.[65] Data from the Centers for Disease Control and Prevention's ABCs program suggested that widespread use of PCV7 has resulted in a 99% decrease in disease caused by vaccine serotypes and serotype 6A, a serotype against which PCV7 provides some cross-protection. PCV7 resulted in 20% fewer episodes of chest radiograph–confirmed pneumonia,[2] 7% fewer episodes of acute otitis media,[66] and 20% fewer tympanostomy tube placements among vaccinated children. PCV7 also reduces nasopharyngeal carriage with pneumococcal vaccine serotypes.[64] As a result of herd protection, decline in the rates of IPD was also observed in unvaccinated persons such as HIV-infected adults, among whom an 88% reduction in vaccine-type IPD was reported in the 7 years after PCV7 introduction for children.[67]

In 2010, a 13-valent conjugate vaccine (PCV13 [Prevnar-13], Pfizer, New York, NY) replaced PCV7. PCV13 includes serotypes 1, 3, 5, 6A, 7F, and19A in addition to the serotypes found in PCV7. These additional serotypes accounting for up to 61% of invasive disease before PCV13 replaced PCV7 in 2010, with 19A causing 43% of the cases.[9] PCV13 was found to elicit similar antibody responses to those against

Table 4
Difference between incidence expected in the absence of PCV13 and that noted after introduction of the vaccine

	2010–11[a]	2011–12[a]	2012–13[a]
≤5 y			
All	−45% (−50 to −40)	−58% (−63 to −53)	−64% (−68 to −59)
PCV13 minus PCV7	−66% (−70 to −61)	−88% (−89 to −86)	−93% (−94 to −91)
Non-PCV13	−4% (−16 to 12)	7% (−9 to 31)	−2% (−19 to 27)
5–17 y			
All	−33% (−45 to −18)	−36% (−49 to −16)	−53% (−64 to −35)
PCV13 minus PCV7	−33% (−45 to −21)	−59% (−66 to −48)	−75% (−80 to −67)
Non-PCV13	−11% (−31 to 25)	32% (−2 to 110)	−2% (−32 to 80)
18–49 y			
All	−12% (−20 to −5)	−37% (−43 to −30)	−32% (−40 to −22)
PCV13 minus PCV7	−33% (−38 to −26)	−64% (−68 to −60)	−72% (−75 to −69)
Non-PCV13	3% (−6 to 15)	−10% (−20 to 4)	13% (−2 to 34)
50–64 y			
All	−8% (−14 to −2)	−28% (−33 to −22)	−18% (−26 to −10)
PCV13 minus PCV7	−23% (−28 to −18)	−54% (−57 to −50)	−62% (−65 to −59)
Non-PCV13	8% (0 to 18)	0% (−9 to 12)	26% (13 to 44)
≥65 y			
All	−6% (−14 to 3)	−19% (−27 to −9)	−12% (−22 to 1)
PCV13 minus PCV7	−23% (−31 to −13)	−46% (−52 to −39)	−58% (−64 to −52)
Non-PCV13	1% (−6 to 10)	−7% (−15 to 3)	7% (−4 to 20)

Data are difference in incidence (95% interval estimate).
[a] July 1 to June 30.
From Moore MR, Link-Gelles R, Schaffner W, et al. Effect of use of 13-valent pneumococcal conjugate vaccine in children on invasive pneumococcal disease in children and adults in the USA: analysis of multisite, population-based surveillance. Lancet Infect Dis 2015;15:523; with permission.

the serotypes contained in PCV7 and induced very robust antibody responses to the 6 additional serotypes in the vaccine. Shortly after its implementation, PCV13 has resulted in dramatic reductions in IPD among children and, through herd protection, among adults.[28,68] Since 2010, incidence of overall IPD in the United States declined by 64%, and IPD caused by an additional 6 serotypes in PCV13 declined by 93% among children younger than 5 years. Among unvaccinated adults, incidence of IPD overall also declined by 12% to 32%, and IPD caused by PCV13 unique serotypes declined by 58% to 72%, depending on age (**Table 4**).[28] A randomized, placebo-controlled trial (CAPiTA trial) among approximately 85,000 vaccinated adults age ≥65 years found 45.6% efficacy of PCV13 against vaccine-type pneumococcal pneumonia, 45.0% efficacy against vaccine-type nonbacteremic pneumococcal pneumonia, and 75.0% efficacy against vaccine-type IPD among adults age ≥65 years.[69] In June 2014, ACIP recommended routine use of both PCV13 and PPSV23 in series to all adults age ≥65 years.[70]

SUMMARY

Universal immunization of infants and toddlers with PCVs over the last 15 years has dramatically altered the landscape of pneumococcal disease. Decreases in IPD, all-cause pneumonia, empyema, mastoiditis, acute otitis media, and complicated otitis media have been reported from multiple countries where universal immunization has been implemented. Introduction of childhood pneumococcal vaccines has also led to expanded understanding of pneumococcal disease: observations have confirmed that most pneumococci are transmitted from children to adults, and that pneumococcal serotypes are not equal in terms of common clinical syndromes, likelihood of antibiotic resistance, or likelihood of progression to disease once colonization occurs. Children with comorbid conditions have higher rates of pneumococcal disease and increased case fatality rates compared with otherwise healthy children, and protection for the most vulnerable pediatric patients will require new strategies to address the underlying host susceptibility and the expanded spectrum of serotypes observed.

REFERENCES

1. Jain S, Williams DJ, Arnold SR, et al. Community-acquired pneumonia requiring hospitalization among U.S. children. N Engl J Med 2015;372:835–45.
2. Griffin M, Zhu Y, Moore M, et al. U.S. hospitalizations for pneumonia after a decade of pneumococcal vaccination. N Engl J Med 2013;369:155–63.
3. Dagan R, Givon-Lavi N, Zamir O, et al. Reduction of nasopharyngeal carriage of Streptococcus pneumoniae after administration of a 9-valent pneumococcal conjugate vaccine to toddlers attending day care centers. J Infect Dis 2002;185:927–36.
4. Granat SM, Mia Z, Ollgren J, et al. Longitudinal study on pneumococcal carriage during the first year of life in Bangladesh. Pediatr Infect Dis J 2007;20.319–24.
5. Ampofo K, Byington C. Streptocccoccus pneumoniae. In: Long SS, Pickering LK, Prober CG, editors. Principles and practice of pediatric infectious diseases. Philadelphia: Churchill Livingstone; 2012. p. 721–8.
6. Gray BM, Converse GM 3rd, Dillon HC Jr. Epidemiologic studies of Streptococcus pneumoniae in infants: acquisition, carriage, and infection during the first 24 months of life. J Infect Dis 1980;142:923–33.
7. Centers for Disease Control and Prevention (CDC). Preventing pneumococcal disease among infants and young children. Recommendations of the Advisory

Committee on Immunization Practices (ACIP). MMWR Morb Mortal Wkly Rep 2000;49:1–35.

8. Yildirim I, Hanage WP, Lipsitch M, et al. Serotype specific invasive capacity and persistent reduction in invasive pneumococcal disease. Vaccine 2010;29:283–8.

9. World Health Organization (WHO). Review of serotype replacement in the setting of 7-valent pneumococcal conjugate vaccine (PCV-7) use and implications for the PCV10/PCV13 era. Geneva (Switzerland): World Health Organization; 2012.

10. Robinson KA, Baughman W, Rothrock G, et al. Epidemiology of invasive Streptococcus pneumoniae infections in the United States, 1995-1998: opportunities for prevention in the conjugate vaccine era. JAMA 2001;285:1729–35.

11. Cherian T, Steinhoff MC, Harrison LH, et al. A cluster of invasive pneumococcal disease in young children in child care. JAMA 1994;271:695–7.

12. Centers for Disease Control and Prevention (CDC). Invasive pneumococcal disease in young children before licensure of 13-valent pneumococcal conjugate vaccine - United States, 2007. MMWR Morb Mortal Wkly Rep 2010;59:253–7.

13. Yildirim I, Stevenson A, Hsu KK, et al. Evolving picture of invasive pneumococcal disease in massachusetts children: a comparison of disease in 2007-2009 with earlier periods. Pediatr Infect Dis J 2012;31:1016–21.

14. Hoffman JA, Mason EO, Schutze GE, et al. Streptococcus pneumoniae infections in the neonate. Pediatrics 2003;112:1095–102.

15. Tsai CJ, Griffin MR, Nuorti JP, et al. Changing epidemiology of pneumococcal meningitis after the introduction of pneumococcal conjugate vaccine in the United States. Clin Infect Dis 2008;46:1664–72.

16. Harboe ZB, Dalby T, Weinberger DM, et al. Impact of 13-valent pneumococcal conjugate vaccination in invasive pneumococcal disease incidence and mortality. Clin Infect Dis 2014;59:1066–73.

17. Centers for Disease Control and Prevention (CDC). Direct and indirect effects of routine vaccination of children with 7-valent pneumococcal conjugate vaccine on incidence of invasive pneumococcal disease-United States, 1998-2003. MMWR Morb Mortal Wkly Rep 2005;54:893–7.

18. Whitney CG, Farley MM, Hadler J, et al. Decline in invasive pneumococcal disease after the introduction of protein-polysaccharide conjugate vaccine. N Engl J Med 2003;348:1737–46.

19. Singleton RJ, Hennessy TW, Bulkow LR, et al. Invasive pneumococcal disease caused by nonvaccine serotypes among alaska native children with high levels of 7-valent pneumococcal conjugate vaccine coverage. JAMA 2007;297: 1784–92.

20. Grall N, Hurmic O, Al Nakib M, et al. Epidemiology of Streptococcus pneumoniae in France before introduction of the PCV-13 vaccine. Eur J Clin Microbiol Infect Dis 2011;30:1511–9.

21. Munoz-Almagro C, Jordan I, Gene A, et al. Emergence of invasive pneumococcal disease caused by nonvaccine serotypes in the era of 7-valent conjugate vaccine. Clin Infect Dis 2008;46:174–82.

22. Grijalva CG, Nuorti JP, Zhu Y, et al. Increasing incidence of empyema complicating childhood community-acquired pneumonia in the United States. Clin Infect Dis 2010;50:805–13.

23. Byington CL, Korgenski K, Daly J, et al. Impact of the pneumococcal conjugate vaccine on pneumococcal parapneumonic empyema. Pediatr Infect Dis J 2006; 25:250–4.

24. Obando I, Arroyo LA, Sanchez-Tatay D, et al. Molecular typing of pneumococci causing parapneumonic empyema in Spanish children using multilocus

sequence typing directly on pleural fluid samples. Pediatr Infect Dis J 2006;25: 962–3.

25. Halgrimson WR, Chan KH, Abzug MJ, et al. Incidence of acute mastoiditis in Colorado children in the pneumococcal conjugate vaccine era. Pediatr Infect Dis J 2014;33:453–7.

26. Bender JM, Ampofo K, Byington CL, et al. Epidemiology of Streptococcus pneumoniae-induced hemolytic uremic syndrome in Utah children. Pediatr Infect Dis J 2010;29:712–6.

27. Lee CF, Liu SC, Lue KH, et al. Pneumococcal pneumonia with empyema and hemolytic uremic syndrome in children: report of three cases. J Microbiol Immunol Infect 2006;39:348–52.

28. Moore MR, Link-Gelles R, Schaffner W, et al. Effect of use of 13-valent pneumococcal conjugate vaccine in children on invasive pneumococcal disease in children and adults in the USA: analysis of multisite, population-based surveillance. Lancet Infect Dis 2015;15:301–9.

29. Pelton SI, Weycker D, Farkouh RA, et al. Risk of pneumococcal disease in children with chronic medical conditions in the era of pneumococcal conjugate vaccine. Clin Infect Dis 2014;59:615–23.

30. Shea KM, Edelsberg J, Weycker D, et al. Rates of pneumococcal disease in adults with chronic medical conditions. Open Forum Infect Dis 2014;1: ofu024.

31. Muhammad RD, Oza-Frank R, Zell E, et al. Epidemiology of invasive pneumococcal disease among high-risk adults since the introduction of pneumococcal conjugate vaccine for children. Clin Infect Dis 2013;56:e59–67.

32. Yildirim I, Shea KM, Little BA, et al, Members of the Massachusetts Department of Public Health. Vaccination, underlying comorbidities, and risk of invasive pneumococcal disease. Pediatrics 2015;135:495–503.

33. Centers for Disease Control and Prevention (CDC). Use of 13-valent pneumococcal conjugate vaccine and 23-valent pneumococcal polysaccharide vaccine for adults with immunocompromising conditions: recommendations of the Advisory Committee on Immunization Practices (ACIP). MMWR Morb Mortal Wkly Rep 2012;61:816–9.

34. O'Brien KL, Moulton LH, Reid R, et al. Efficacy and safety of seven-valent conjugate pneumococcal vaccine in American Indian children: group randomised trial. Lancet 2003;362:355–61.

35. van Hoek AJ, Andrews N, Waight PA, et al. The effect of underlying clinical conditions on the risk of developing invasive pneumococcal disease in England. J Infect 2012;65:17–24.

36. Inghammar M, Engstrom G, Kahlmeter G, et al. Invasive pneumococcal disease in patients with an underlying pulmonary disorder. Clin Microbiol Infect 2013;19: 1148–54.

37. Reefhuis J, Honein MA, Whitney CG, et al. Risk of bacterial meningitis in children with cochlear implants. N Engl J Med 2003;349:435–45.

38. Talbot TR, Hartert TV, Mitchel E, et al. Asthma as a risk factor for invasive pneumococcal disease. N Engl J Med 2005;352:2082–90.

39. Ladhani SN, Slack MP, Andrews NJ, et al. Invasive pneumococcal disease after routine pneumococcal conjugate vaccination in children, England and Wales. Emerg Infect Dis 2013;19:61–8.

40. Ladhani SN, Andrews NJ, Waight P, et al. Invasive pneumococcal disease, comorbidities, and polysaccharide vaccine use in children aged 5-15 years in England and Wales. Clin Infect Dis 2014;58:517–25.

41. Rosenow EC. Studies in pneumonia and pneumococcus infection. J Infect Dis 2004;189:132–64.
42. Coant PN, Kornberg AE, Duffy LC, et al. Blood culture results as determinants in the organism identification of bacterial meningitis. Pediatr Emerg Care 1992;8:200–5.
43. Neuman MI, Harper MB. Evaluation of a rapid urine antigen assay for the detection of invasive pneumococcal disease in children. Pediatrics 2003;112:1279–82.
44. Marcos MA, Martinez E, Almela M, et al. New rapid antigen test for diagnosis of pneumococcal meningitis. Lancet 2001;357:1499–500.
45. Saha SK, Darmstadt GL, Yamanaka N, et al. Rapid diagnosis of pneumococcal meningitis: implications for treatment and measuring disease burden. Pediatr Infect Dis J 2005;24:1093–8.
46. Murdoch DR. Molecular genetic methods in the diagnosis of lower respiratory tract infections. APMIS 2004;112:713–27.
47. Tzanakaki G, Tsopanomichalou M, Kesanopoulos K, et al. Simultaneous single-tube PCR assay for the detection of Neisseria meningitidis, Haemophilus influenzae type b and Streptococcus pneumoniae. Clin Microbiol Infect 2005;11:386–90.
48. Seng P, Rolain JM, Fournier PE, et al. MALDI-TOF-mass spectrometry applications in clinical microbiology. Future Microbiol 2010;5:1733–54.
49. Vernet G, Saha S, Satzke C, et al. Laboratory-based diagnosis of pneumococcal pneumonia: state of the art and unmet needs. Clin Microbiol Infect 2011;17(Suppl 3):1–13.
50. Martinez RM, Bauerle ER, Fang FC, et al. Evaluation of three rapid diagnostic methods for direct identification of microorganisms in positive blood cultures. J Clin Microbiol 2014;52:2521–9.
51. Available at: http://www.accessdata.fda.gov/cdrh_docs/reviews/K130914.pdf. Accessed July 27, 2015.
52. Altun O, Almuhayawi M, Ullberg M, et al. Rapid identification of microorganisms from sterile body fluids by use of FilmArray. J Clin Microbiol 2015;53:710–2.
53. Werno AM, Murdoch DR. Medical microbiology: laboratory diagnosis of invasive pneumococcal disease. Clin Infect Dis 2008;46:926–32.
54. Vuori-Holopainen E, Salo E, Saxen H, et al. Etiological diagnosis of childhood pneumonia by use of transthoracic needle aspiration and modern microbiological methods. Clin Infect Dis 2002;34:583–90.
55. Tunkel AR, Hartman BJ, Kaplan SL, et al. Practice guidelines for the management of bacterial meningitis. Clin Infect Dis 2004;39:1267–84.
56. Le J, Bradley JS, Murray W, et al. Improved vancomycin dosing in children using area under the curve exposure. Pediatr Infect Dis J 2013;32:e155–63.
57. Pelton SI, Jacobs MR. Pneumococcal infections. In: Cherry JD, Harrision GJ, Kaplan SL, editors. Feigin and Cherry's textbook of pediatric infectious diseases. 7th edition. Philadelphia: Elsevier Saunders; 2014. p. 1198–246.
58. Committee on Infectious Diseases American Academy of Pediatrics. Pneumococcal infections. In: Kimberlin DW, Brady MT, Jackson MA, et al, editors. Report of the Committee on Infectious Diseases. 30th edition. Elk Grove Village (IL): American Academy of Pediatrics; 2015. p. 638–44.
59. Schut ES, Brouwer MC, de Gans J, et al. Delayed cerebral thrombosis after initial good recovery from pneumococcal meningitis. Neurology 2009;73:1988–95.
60. Weinstein MP, Klugman KP, Jones RN. Rationale for revised penicillin susceptibility breakpoints versus Streptococcus pneumoniae: coping with antimicrobial susceptibility in an era of resistance. Clin Infect Dis 2009;48:1596–600.

61. Jackson LA, Neuzil KM. Pneumococcal polysaccharide vaccine. In: Plotkin SA, Orenstein WA, Offit PA, editors. Vaccines. 5th edition. Philadelphia: Elsevier Saunders; 2008. p. 569–604.
62. Sanders LA, Rijkers GT, Kuis W, et al. Defective antipneumococcal polysaccharide antibody response in children with recurrent respiratory tract infections. J Allergy Clin Immunol 1993;91:110–9.
63. Centers for Disease Control and Prevention (CDC). Prevention of pneumococcal disease among infants and children: use of 13-valent pneumococcal conjugate vaccine and 23-valent pneumococcal polysaccharide vaccine: recommendations of the Advisory Committee on Immunization Practices (ACIP). MMWR Morb Mortal Wkly Rep 2010;59:1–18.
64. Black S, Shinefield H, Fireman B, et al. Efficacy, safety and immunogenicity of heptavalent pneumococcal conjugate vaccine in children. Northern California Kaiser Permanente Vaccine Study Center Group. Pediatr Infect Dis J 2000;19: 187–95.
65. World Health Organization (WHO). Pneumococcal conjugate vaccine for childhood immunization-WHO position paper. Wkly Epidemiol Rec 2007;12:93–104.
66. Grijalva C, Poehling K, Nuorti J, et al. National impact of universal childhood immunization with pneumococcal conjugate vaccine on outpatient medical care visits in the United States. Pediatrics 2006;118:865–73.
67. Cohen A, Harrison L, Farley M, et al. Prevention of invasive pneumococcal disease among HIV-infected adults in the era of childhood pneumococcal immunization. AIDS 2010;24:2253–62.
68. Kaplan S, Barson W, Lin P, et al. Early trends for invasive pneumococcal infections in children after the introduction of the 13-valent pneumococcal conjugate vaccine. Pediatr Infect Dis J 2013;32:203–7.
69. Bonten M, Huijts S, Bolkenbaas M, et al. Polysaccharide Conjugate Vaccine against Pneumococcal Pneumonia in Adults. N Engl J Med 2015;372:1114–25.
70. Centers for Disease Control and Prevention (CDC). Use of 13-Valent Pneumococcal Conjugate Vaccine and 23-Valent Pneumococcal Polysaccharide Vaccine Among Adults Aged ≥65 years: recommendations of the Advisory Committee on Immunization Practices (ACIP). MMWR Morb Mortal Wkly Rep 2014;63:822–5.

Pertussis in the Era of New Strains of *Bordetella pertussis*

Emily Souder, MD*, Sarah S. Long, MD

KEYWORDS

- *Bordetella pertussis* • Waning immunity • Whole-cell vaccine • Acellular vaccine
- Strain adaptation

KEY POINTS

- Incidence of pertussis has increased since the 1980s with the most recent outbreaks reaching the highest number of cases in 60 years.
- Recent outbreaks in the United States show increasing number of cases among fully vaccinated children and adolescents, suggesting rapidly waning immunity after administration of acellular pertussis vaccines.
- Adaption by the pathogen, likely from vaccine pressure, has led to the divergence of vaccine strains from circulating strains.
- Maternal vaccination during each pregnancy is the best strategy currently to prevent severe morbidity and mortality from pertussis in young infants.

ETIOLOGY, TRANSMISSION, AND VIRULENCE

Bordetella pertussis, a fastidious, tiny, gram-negative coccobacillus is the cause of epidemic pertussis and most cases of sporadic pertussis.[1–5] Several *Bordetella* species, including *Bordetella parapertussis*, *Bordetella bronchiseptica*, and *Bordetella holmesii*, can cause respiratory illness. Although *B pertussis* is found only in humans, other species are found in animals, including dogs, cats, and rabbits, and *B bronchiseptica* can cause disease such as kennel cough in dogs.[6]

Pertussis is highly contagious and is transmitted via aerosolized droplets through close contact during coughing or sneezing. Studies have identified household members as the source in 75% of cases in infants, mothers being the likely source in almost

Neither Dr S.S. Long nor Dr E. Souder has a conflict of interest to disclose.
Dr E. Souder wrote the first draft of the article.
Section of Infectious Diseases, Department of Pediatrics, St. Christopher's Hospital for Children, Drexel University College of Medicine, 160 East Erie Avenue, Philadelphia, PA 19134, USA
* Corresponding author.
E-mail address: Emily.souder@drexelmed.edu

Infect Dis Clin N Am 29 (2015) 699–713
http://dx.doi.org/10.1016/j.idc.2015.07.005
0891-5520/15/\$ – see front matter © 2015 Elsevier Inc. All rights reserved.
id.theclinics.com

one-half of these cases.[7] Other risk factors for infants include large households, especially if there are siblings older than 6 years.[8]

B pertussis has many virulence factors, several antigens of which are represented in current vaccines. Many of these can be characterized as toxins or adhesins. The exact mechanism of cough illness is unknown. Pertussis toxin disrupts function in many cell types and also causes lymphocytosis by inhibiting their regression from the vasculature.[9,10] Pertussis toxin, once thought to be the molecule causing pertussis, has since been found to be important but not essential. Filamentous hemagglutinin, pertactin, and fimbriae are important for adhesion of *B pertussis* to respiratory tract epithelium. Pertactin also interferes with the pathogen's opsonophagocytosis by neutrophils.[10–12] Adenylate cyclase toxin also can inhibit phagocyte function and causes apoptosis of host cells. Tracheal cytotoxin is cidal to respiratory tract epithelial cells in vitro.[10] Inactivated pertussis toxin, filamentous hemagglutinin, and pertactin, with or without fimbriae, are present in currently available US acellular pertussis vaccines.

EPIDEMIOLOGY

Although pertussis was first recognized in the Middle Ages, *B pertussis* was not isolated and identified as the cause until 1906. The first known epidemic of pertussis occurred in 1578 in Paris, and since then endemic infection as well as cyclic outbreaks of pertussis have continued throughout the world.[1,13] Worldwide there are an estimated 16 million cases of pertussis and 195,000 deaths in children annually.[14] **Fig. 1** shows the numbers of cases and introduction of vaccines over time in the United States. Before implementation of routine vaccination in the United States, pertussis was an inescapable part of childhood, with hundreds of thousands of cases annually and an average annual attack rate of greater than 150 cases per 100,000 individuals from 1932 to 1941.[15–17] In 1934, greater than 260,000 cases of pertussis were reported, the highest annual incidence ever recorded.[18] In 1940, the diphtheria and tetanus toxoids and whole-cell pertussis vaccine (DPT or DTP) first became available and was recommended by the American Academy of Pediatrics (AAP) for routine use in children in 1943.[2] After introduction of DTP in the United States, there was a 100-fold decline in incidence of pertussis by the 1970s, reaching a nadir of 1010 cases in 1976.[15,18] However, unlike other diseases such as measles and varicella, neither infection nor immunization produces lifelong immunity against pertussis, and there continue to be cyclical peaks in incidence every 2 to 5 years.[16,18,19] Historically, the

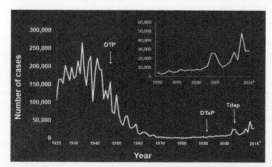

Fig. 1. Pertussis cases reported in the United States in the National Notifiable Diseases Surveillance System, 1922–2014. [a]2014 data are provisional. (*From* CDC, National Notifiable Diseases Surveillance System and Supplemental Pertussis Surveillance System and 1922–1949, passive reports to the Public Health Service.)

incidence of pertussis decreased with increasing age; however, in the 1980s (during use of DTP vaccines), a steady increase in the number of reported pertussis cases began, with a shift in prevalence to young adolescents by the 1990s[1] (**Fig. 2**). Meanwhile, due to reactogenicity of DTP and concerns about vaccine-associated potential adverse central nervous system effects, DTPs were replaced by acellular pertussis vaccines (DTaPs) for the reinforcing fourth and fifth doses in 1992 and then to include the infant primary series in 1997.[2,20,21]

Increasing pertussis in adolescents continued in the early 2000s, and in 2004, an epidemic year, adolescents comprised 30% of all cases.[2] That same year the CDC and the AAP recommended a booster dose of tetanus toxoid–reduced diphtheria toxoid–acellular pertussis vaccine (Tdap) for 11- to 12-year-olds to reduce the burden of disease in adolescence.[2,22,23] Although universal use of Tdap was successful in decreasing disease in the adolescent age group, there was no community (herd) protection accrued to infants. There then followed another notable change in epidemiology. From 2007 to 2009, reported cases among 7- to 10-year-olds, a group previously considered at low risk, increased disproportionately from 13% to 23% of reported cases. These children were in the first birth cohort to have received acellular pertussis vaccine for the entire infant and preschool series.[24]

In 2010, an epidemic of pertussis in California included more than 9000 cases reported and 10 infant deaths, the highest in 60 years.[25] Although the highest age-related incidence was among infants younger than 1 year, there was an increased rate among 7- to 10-year-olds, most of whom were fully vaccinated. Several other states reported epidemic levels of pertussis in 2012, with greater than 48,000 cases nationwide, the highest recorded since 1955.[11] Washington, one of the states with epidemic levels, reported 2520 cases by June 2012, an increase of 1300% from the prior year.[26] Although infants younger than 1 year and 10-year-olds continued to have the highest incidence of disease, a new age-related increase occurred among 13- to 14 year-olds, a cohort recently vaccinated with Tdap.[26] A similar epidemiologic pattern has occurred throughout the United States, suggesting rapidly waning immunity after administration of acellular pertussis vaccines. The most recent epidemic in California in 2014 accrued more cases than in 2010, with peak incidence in infants and 14- to 16-year-olds.[27]

The reason for the increased incidence of pertussis in the last several decades likely is related to several overlapping and sequential factors: enhanced awareness by physicians, increased detection through newer methods such as polymerase chain reaction (PCR) testing, lower effectiveness of acellular vaccines compared with potent whole-cell vaccines, return to susceptibility quickly with waning of DTaP and Tdap

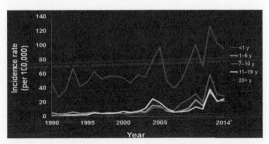

Fig. 2. Pertussis incidence by age group reported in the United States, 1990–2014. [a]2014 data are provisional. (*From* CDC, National Notifiable Diseases Surveillance System and Supplemental Pertussis Surveillance System.)

vaccine-induced antibody, increase in groups of unvaccinated children, and genetic changes in the pathogen (**Fig. 3**).[4,5,28]

Role of Waning Immunity in Current Epidemiology

Short-term vaccine efficacy after the fifth dose of DTaP may be as high as 98% within the first year, but protection decreases rapidly. A meta-analysis estimated only 10% protection by 8.5 years after the fifth dose.[9,25,28] In the 2010 California epidemic, increased risk of disease occurred with time since the fifth dose of DTaP, with the highest incidence in the 10-year-old cohort (whose primary series was solely acellular vaccine). The odds of developing pertussis after the fifth dose of DTaP was 1.42 per year or an increased odds of infection of 42% each year.[29] Vaccine effectiveness in 8- to 12-year-olds has been estimated to be only 24%.[30] Rates and risk ratios of pertussis were analyzed in children in recent outbreaks in Oregon and Minnesota. Likelihood of pertussis after the fifth dose of DTaP increased rapidly with risk ratios of 1.9 at year 2 and 8.9 at year 6 after immunization.[24] Rapidly waning immunity after DTaP also has been seen in other countries. In Australia, the fourth dose of acellular vaccine was discontinued for children at 18 months in 2003. At present, 3-year-olds have a greater risk of pertussis than infants.[3]

The effectiveness and duration of protection following Tdap administration also has come under scrutiny. In a cohort of Wisconsin residents born between 1998 and 2000, decreasing Tdap effectiveness was found with increasing time since vaccination. Tdap effectiveness less than 1 year after vaccination was 75.3% but declined to 11.9% by 3 to 4 years postvaccination.[22]

In the 2010 California and 2012 Washington state outbreaks, the risk of pertussis was remarkably lower among older adolescents who likely had received at least 1 dose of DTP in infancy, suggesting a superior, boostable protective effect of even distant priming with whole-cell vaccine (DTP).[26,29] In a study of children in a large health care system in California, individuals who had received all 5 doses of DTaP had an 8.57 relative risk of pertussis compared with those who had received at least 1 dose of DTP. Although increased risk after DTaPs administration could be partially mitigated by a Tdap booster, protection was enhanced in individuals who had ever received whole-cell vaccine.[31]

Differences between the immunizing antigens, process of pertussis toxin deactivation, as well as adjuvants in whole-cell and acellular vaccines likely contribute to their sustainable effectiveness. Whole-cell vaccine contains inactivated *B pertussis*

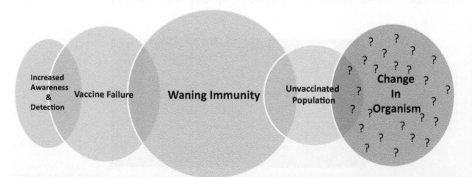

Fig. 3. Potential relative importance of multiple factors likely associated with current high incidence of pertussis.

bacteria, while acellular vaccines contain a combination of 1 to 5 purified pertussis proteins: inactivated pertussis toxin, pertactin, filamentous hemagglutinin, and fimbriae types 2 and 3.[32] DTP and DTaP elicit different immunologic responses. Both vaccines induce a T_H2 humoral response that stimulates B lymphocytes to produce antibodies that are protective against disease short term. Although high level of antibodies are elicited after administration of acellular vaccines, the range is narrow, that is, only to purified antigens included in the vaccine.[9] Whole-cell vaccines also elicit a T_H1-cell-mediated response, simulating natural infection. Cellular response contributes to protection through macrophage activation and intracellular killing of *B pertussis*, an important aspect of control and clearance of pertussis.[3,33] Absent cellular immunity, susceptibility to infection returns more immediately after administration of acellular pertussis vaccines when antibody begins to wane and at higher antibody levels compared with whole-cell vaccines.

Role of Strain Adaptation in Current Epidemiology

The typical narrow immune response following administration of acellular vaccines likely favors the selection of escape mutants of *B pertussis*.[1,32] Pathogen adaptation since the introduction of the acellular vaccines likely also plays a role in the current surge of pertussis. Divergence of circulating strains from vaccine strains, however, began during the DTP era, the first genetic adaptations occurring through allelic changes of surface proteins (pertussis toxin, pertactin, fimbriae).[9,34] These changes affected structure or regulation, such as upregulation of expression of toxins. Allelic changes leading to divergence of circulating strains from US vaccine strains are shown in **Table 1**. Such allelic changes were not associated consistently with increased notifications of pertussis in the United States.

Acellular vaccines licensed in the United States contain a combination of purified protein components, including inactivated pertussis toxin, pertactin, and filamentous hemagglutinin. One manufacturer's vaccines also contain 2 fimbrial proteins.[35] These vaccines were developed to mirror the alleles of predominant *B pertussis* strains of previous decades as well as those included in DTPs. The molecular profiles using multilocus variable number tandem repeat analysis (MLVA) for the 2 strains used in currently licensed vaccines are *prn1-ptxA2-ptxP1-fim3A* (Tohama I) and *prn1-ptxA4-ptxP1-fim3A* (strain 10536). Other countries use vaccines with different combinations of alleles.[9,35,36] Many investigators suggest that the minimal impact of vaccination on *B pertussis* colonization, together with the lack of cellular immune response to acellular vaccines, favors selection of escape mutants at antibody waning.

Fimbriae

Both *fim2* and *fim3* are present in *B pertussis*, of which one or both genes can be expressed with alleles exhibiting little overall variation.[9] A US study of pertussis isolates from 1935 to 2009 first noted a new fimbrial allele in 1994, *fim3B*. The *fim3B* allele has become the predominant allele in circulating *B pertussis* strains in the US and also

Table 1
Antigenic alleles in current acellular pertussis vaccines compared with current circulating *B pertussis* strains

Vaccine Strains	Circulating Strains
prn1-ptxA2-ptxP1-fim3A	*prn2-ptxA1-ptxP3-fim3A/B*
prn1-ptxA4-ptxP1-fim3A	—

has coincided with increased notifications of pertussis.[36] In the pertussis outbreak in Washington state in 2012, *fim3A* reemerged and became predominant, an event that has not occurred since the early 2000s.[37] In the Netherlands, however, where there was an increase in *fim3B* allele during a similar period as in the United States, there was not a direct correlation with notifications of pertussis. It is possible that the impact of fimbrial mutations could differ depending on the acellular vaccine in use.[36]

Pertussis toxin

Pertussis toxin comprises 5 subunits. *PtxA* has the most potent toxic activity and is the most immunogenic of the group. The *ptxA* subunit has several allelic variants of which *ptxA2* and *ptxA4* are present in strains used to derive many acellular vaccines, including those used in the United States and Europe.[1,9] A study of *B pertussis* strains circulating in several European countries between 1998 and 2012 found the most common *ptxA* allele to be a nonvaccine type allele *ptxA1*.[32] Similarly, a comparison of allelic frequencies in circulating strains between 1990 and 2004 in 4 countries using whole-cell vaccines (Argentina, Finland, Russia, and the United Kingdom) showed that 100% of clinical isolates contained *ptxA1*, suggesting that antigenic divergence from vaccine strains occurred globally and regardless of vaccine type.[1]

A mutation in the regulator gene for pertussis toxin also has occurred. The pertussis toxin promoter gene (*ptxP*) is a major virulence factor. Multiple alleles for *ptxP* are described of which *ptxP1*, *ptxP2*, and *ptxP3* are predominant worldwide. A recent increase in the *ptxP3* allele in the Netherlands has been associated temporally with an increase in the number of pertussis cases.[1] Although *ptxP3* largely has replaced the *ptxP1* allele worldwide (including in the United States), with some countries reporting 90% of strains carrying *ptxP3*, a direct correlation with increased incidence of pertussis has been inconsistent.[9,36] The allele for *ptxP3* is associated with 1.6 times greater production of pertussis toxin compared with *ptxP1* strains, suggesting increased fitness related to the mutation.[38] A study in the Netherlands correlated the temporal epidemiologic increase in *ptxP3* to increased incidences of pertussis hospitalization and deaths.[38] However, the *ptxP* allele was not characterized in this study.[1,36] Profound lymphocytosis and subsequent pulmonary hypertension in infants, an indirect measure of pertussis toxin level, has been associated with death.[9,10] Increased toxin production associated with the *ptxP3* allele also may exert an advantage in vaccinated hosts by delaying an effective immune response, thus allowing for enhanced transmission.[9] Complement plays an important role in *B pertussis* killing. It has been discovered that strains with the *ptxP3* allele, compared with other *ptxP* alleles, produce higher amounts of a complement evasion protein, autotransporter Vag8, supporting the theory of increased fitness of *B pertussis* containing *ptxP3*.[39]

Pertactin

Several pertactin protein alleles are identified, including *prn1*, *prn2*, *prn3*, and *prn13*. In several European countries, *prn2* now predominates with a frequency of 99%.[32] In the United States, *prn2* has predominated since the 1990s, and in a series of 60 *B pertussis* isolates from a US hospital, greater than 98% of strains had the *prn2* allele.[40,41] The oldest UK and US *B pertussis* strains isolated from 1920 and 1935, respectively, express *prn1*. The dominance of *prn2* likely arose during DTP pressure. Strains from a largely unvaccinated population in Africa in the 1990s contained *prn1*.[1]

Recent and dramatic *B pertussis* mutations have resulted in pertactin deficiency. This deficiency has occurred rapidly and through multiple mechanisms. Unlike allelic changes that occurred during universal use of whole-cell vaccines, pertactin deficiency has occurred more dramatically and only during exclusive use of acellular vaccines. Pertactin-deficient strains have emerged in many countries worldwide, including France, Japan, Australia, Finland, Italy, and the United States, where acellular vaccines have been implemented. In the United States, pertactin-deficient strains were first identified in Philadelphia[40] and subsequently shown that among 1300 isolates from 1934 to 2009 collected by the CDC from surveillance studies and outbreaks, the first pertactin-deficient strain was isolated in 1994.[35] In a Philadelphia collection, the first pertactin-deficient strain was isolated in 2008 and has increased each year with an overall prevalence of 68% during the period from 2007 to 2014.[41] In the CDC collection, after a single pertactin-deficient isolate in 1994, the next was found only among 2010 isolates,[35] with a rapid increase thereafter with pertactin-deficient strains accounting for 85% of isolates from 2011 to 2013.[11] In countries such as Poland that continue to use whole-cell vaccine, pertactin-deficient strains have not been found.[5] The prevalence of pertactin-deficient isolates in other countries also has increased rapidly, representing about 78% of Australian isolates and 32% of Japanese isolates currently.[37,42] A variety of mutations leading to loss of pertactin have been identified, including IS481 insertions at multiple locations, premature stop codons and deletions.[35] The high number and diversity of mechanisms and mutations of pertactin loss found throughout the world where acellular pertussis vaccines are used suggest multiple genetic events in multiple strains and a selective advantage of that absence of pertactin expression.[11] Although pertactin is believed to play a role in adherence to respiratory epithelium, a mouse model showed that both pertactin-producing and pertactin-deficient strains were able to colonize mouse lungs similarly. The study also showed that pertactin-deficient strains were able to sustain longer infection and colonization.[34] In the recent epidemic in Washington in 2012, 76% of isolates were pertactin-deficient. Given that most cases occurred in vaccinated children pertactin-deficient strains may have particular advantage in this population.[37] Pertussis is a well-adapted pathogen and may only require small genetic changes to persist and surge in vaccinated populations with waning antibody levels.[9]

CLINICAL FEATURES

Pertussis causes a cough illness in unimmunized or distantly immunized individuals with symptoms typically starting 5 to 10 days after exposure. **Fig. 4** shows clinical courses of pertussis by age and immunization status. In unimmunized children, the

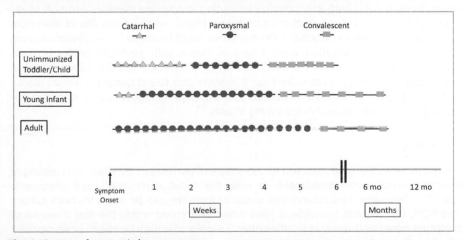

Fig. 4. Stages of pertussis by age group.

illness is characterized by three 2-week stages: catarrhal stage, consisting of symptoms indistinguishable from a minor upper respiratory tract infection with minimal or absent fever; paroxysmal stage, named for its characteristic cough consisting of intermittent, sudden bursts of cough, followed by whoop on inspiration and posttussive emesis; and convalescent stage, when paroxysms wane in number and severity. Patients are most contagious during the catarrhal stage. The paroxysmal stage usually lasts 1 to 6 weeks but can be as long as 10 weeks. The paroxysms of cough are rapid and numerous, occurring up to 15 times in a 24-hour period. The frequency increases during the first few weeks, peaks, and then gradually declines.[43] Although symptoms can be prolonged, there is no evidence for chronic infection or long-term carriage of B pertussis.[10] Paroxysms can recur with subsequent respiratory illnesses months after initial illness and are not associated with recurrent isolation of B pertussis.[6]

Young infants have a short incubation period and frequently come to medical attention because of apnea or gagging, gasping, and choking. Infants younger than 6 months are at highest risk for severe disease and hospitalization, and in the United States, infants younger than 4 months account for greater than 90% of pertussis-related deaths.[44,45] Severe complications in infants include seizures and encephalopathy related to hypoxia, secondary bacterial pneumonia, and pulmonary hypertension.[10]

Adolescents and adults frequently have disease that may not be recognized as pertussis. Whoop is uncommon, but paroxysms of cough and posttussive emesis are common manifestations. A study of adolescents and adults with prolonged cough illness found that 13% to 20% had infection with B pertussis.[16] Pertussis leads to hospitalization in older children and adolescents in only about 1% to 7% of those affected. Among adults, people older than 65 years are at the highest risk of pertussis hospitalization.[46] Complications also are uncommon in adults, occurring in about 5%, but can include syncope, rib fractures, pneumonia, and otitis media.[6,10]

Allelic mutations in virulence proteins of B pertussis have not been consistently associated with enhanced severity of pertussis. Recent studies have compared the clinical manifestations of children with pertussis caused by pertactin-producing versus pertactin-deficient strains. In a French study using pediatrician questionnaires regarding infants younger than 6 months, similar courses of illness were found except for a longer lag between development of cough and hospitalization in those with pertactin-deficient B pertussis, possibly indicating less severe disease.[47] In a US study of 60 patients with culture-confirmed pertussis (most cases <4 months of age) from 2007 to 2014 at a single hospital in Pennsylvania, no differences in the clinical courses and rates of hospitalization were found in those with pertactin-producing and pertactin-deficient strains.[41] The CDC recently characterized 753 B pertussis isolates, predominately from patients older than 6 months and found generally similar illness courses in health department notification forms except for higher rate of reports of apnea in patients with pertactin-producing strains.[11]

DIAGNOSIS

Culture remains the gold standard for diagnosis of pertussis; however, PCR testing of nasopharyngeal swab specimens is now the most commonly used diagnostic test.[48–50] The same nasopharyngeal swab or aspirate can be used for both culture and PCR. Culture has the highest yield when performed within the first 2 weeks of symptom onset and rarely is positive after 3 weeks of cough illness.[20] Unimmunized infants with pertussis almost always have positive results in both tests. Older, previously immunized people and those with cough illness for 2 weeks or more have positive results in either test in less than 20% of cases.

Testing by PCR is more sensitive than culture and can occasionally detect pertussis DNA beyond 3 weeks of illness. Although in one study test-positive cases had a median of 58 days of symptoms after illness onset, PCR probably is most reliable at 4 weeks or less. Beyond 4 weeks, PCR may detect nonviable organisms and the patient may no longer be contagious despite a positive PCR result.[51] Many real-time PCR assays detect IS481, an insertion sequence with multiple copies found in *B pertussis* (218–239 copies) and fewer copies in *B holmesii* (32–65 copies).[49] If IS481 is the only PCR target, testing does not distinguish between *B pertussis* and *B holmesii* nor does it detect *B parapertussis*. Optimizing PCR by inclusion of additional targets, such as IS1001, in assays is required to detect and differentiate species.

For individuals being evaluated beyond 2 weeks of symptoms, serologic tests using enzyme immunoassay to detect antibody against *B pertussis* proteins is most useful.[6] These tests can be performed up to 12 weeks after cough onset. Of commercially available assays, IgG anti–pertussis toxin is the most useful. Generally an antibody level greater than or equal to 90 EU/mL is highly suggestive of pertussis.

Several methods are used to differentiate among strains of *B pertussis*, which is important in determining strain relatedness in outbreaks, and to investigate strain origin and evolution. These methods include pulsed-field gel electrophoresis, MLVA, multiantigen sequence typing, and whole-genome sequencing, which is the gold standard but not practical given its high cost.[37,52] Using these techniques, diversity of pertactin-deficient strains was recognized even within single geographic areas and outbreaks, suggesting multiple independent mutations rather than spread of a single clone. In a recent study analyzing a new typing method, single nucleotide primer extension (SNPeX) was highly discriminating. SNPeX is based on single nucleotide polymorphisms and does not require target DNA PCR amplification. This method is inexpensive and rapid, making it a promising tool for studying strains during outbreaks.[52]

TREATMENT

Antibiotic therapy is recommended for confirmed or suspected pertussis within 6 weeks of symptom onset in infants <1 year of age and within 21 days of onset in older children and adults. Therapy reduces contagiousness and can decrease the severity and duration of symptoms if given in catarrhal/early paroxysmal stages.[43] Postexposure prophylaxis should be provided to healthcare professionals (regardless of immunization status) who have unprotected close exposure to patients with pertussis, especially if they will have contact with other patients or other children at high risk of severe pertussis. Household or other close contacts of people with pertussis also should receive chemoprophylaxis. Intense close contacts in school, i.e. that simulate household exposure, should be considered for PEP. Public health officials should be consulted when considering PEP for a large number of school contacts. Macrolides including azithromycin, clarithromycin and erythromycin remain the mainstay of treatment and prophylaxis in all age groups, with similar dosing for treatment and postexposure prophylaxis. Erythromycin is not recommended for infants <1 month because of association with infantile hypertrophic pyloric stenosis (IHPS), which appears to be higher than with azithromycin.[53,54] A retrospective cohort study of 1,074,236 children from 2001 to 2012 cared for in a military health system found increased risk of IHPS with exposure to erythromycin (adjusted odds ratio

13.3; 95% CI, 6.80-25.9) and azithromycin (adjusted odds ratio 8.26; 95% CI, 2.62–26.0) in the first 14 days of life.[55] Prophylaxis with azithromycin should always be given to young infants exposed to pertussis. Trimethoprim-sulfamethoxazole is an alternative treatment option in those who are not neonates and are unable to take macrolide antibiotics or rarely for a macrolide-resistant strain (**Table 2**).[43]

Supportive care is a critical aspect of hospital management, especially in young infants with apnea associated with paroxysms or respiratory failure. Corticosteroids therapy and intravenous immunoglobulin are not beneficial.[56] Pulmonary hypertension is the usual cause of death in young infants and should be expectantly evaluated. There are several case reports of affected infants surviving after treatment with leukopheresis or exchange transfusion[57]; extracorporeal membrane oxygenation is associated with 90% or more fatality.

PREVENTION STRATEGIES

Full implementation of use of currently available acellular pertussis vaccines is the best means to curtail pertussis.[58] Vaccination reduces contagiousness and severity of disease. In one study in France, vaccination was protective against severe disease, including intensive care unit admission regardless of the strain type.[33,42] In Oregon from 2010 to 2012, vaccinated and unvaccinated children and adolescents with

Table 2
Recommended antimicrobial agents for treatment and postexposure prophylaxis of pertussis

| Agents | Age Group | | | |
	<1 mo	1–5 mo	≥6 mo & Children	Adults
First-line agents				
Azithromycin	Recommended agent, 10 mg/kg once daily × 5 d	10 mg/kg once daily × 5 d	10 mg/kg (max 500 mg) once on day 1; then 5 mg/kg (max 250 mg) once on days 2–5	500 mg once on day 1; then 250 mg once on days 2–5
Clarithromycin	Not recommended	15 mg/kg/d divided bid × 7 d	15 mg/kg/d (max 1 g/d) divided bid × 7 d	1 g/d divided bid × 7 d
Erythromycin	Not preferred	40–50 mg/kg/d divided qid × 14 d	40–50 mg/kg/d (max 2 g/d) divided qid × 14 d	2 g/d divided qid × 14 d
Alternative agents				
TMP-SMX	Contraindicated	Contraindicated at <2 mo. At ≥2 mo, TMP 8 mg/kg/d, SMX 40 mg/kg/d divided bid × 14 d	TMP 8 mg/kg/d, SMX 40 mg/kg/d (max TMP 320 mg/d) divided bid × 14 d	TMP 320 mg, SMX 1600 mg/d divided bid × 14 d

Abbreviations: SMX, sulfamethoxazole; TMP, trimethoprim.
From Tiwari T, Murphy TV, Moran J, National Immunization Program, CDC. Recommended antimicrobial agents for the treatment and postexposure prophylaxis of pertussis: 2005 CDC Guidelines. MMWR Recomm Rep 2005;54(RR-14):1–16.

pertussis were compared. Vaccinated people had decreased illness severity and duration of symptoms, even if not fully vaccinated.[59] In another recent study of fatal and nonfatal pertussis reported nationally from 1991 to 2008, 1 or more doses of DTaP given to infants at greater than or equal to 42 days was protective against pneumonia, hospitalization, and death.[60] Infants should be vaccinated at 6 weeks of age in outbreak settings. Because pertussis is highly contagious, 92% to 95% of the population must be vaccinated to affect transmission.[19] Providers must confidently and unambiguously encourage immunization with DTaP in infants and children and Tdap in adolescents and adults.

With only short-term protection afforded by currently available vaccines, efforts must be focused on protection of the most vulnerable age group, that is, infants too young to be vaccinated. The idea of cocooning was an attractive strategy based on studies showing that about 75% of infants acquire infection from household members.[7] In 2006, the CDC recommended targeted vaccination of postpartum women and all adults in close contact with infants.[8] It has been estimated that such cocooning would result in a 50% decrease in incidence of severe pertussis in infants; however, there have been conflicting outcome studies and limited supporting data. In a Texas study using enhanced attempts to immunize mothers postpartum, there was no decrease in infant hospitalization.[61] An additional study of effect of vaccination of all close contacts of infants younger than 6 months found no reduction in infant illness.[7] One study from Australia found a 51% reduced risk of infant pertussis if the parents were vaccinated. This study identified mothers as the most important source of infection for infants and no independent protective effect by immunizing fathers.[8] Overall, these programs have proved difficult to implement without high resource utilization and are insufficient as a single strategy especially given that infants would be entirely reliant on the immunity of all those around them.[62]

In 2011, the CDC recommended that pregnant women be vaccinated with Tdap during pregnancy if not previously immunized with Tdap. The ideal timing to vaccinate pregnant women is between 27 and 36 weeks' gestation to maximize active transfer of maternal IgG antibodies to the infant.[63,64] A study of the safety and immunogenicity of Tdap in the third trimester of pregnancy found that infants born to vaccinated mothers had substantially higher concentrations of pertussis antibodies at birth and 2 months of age compared with infants born to mothers immunized postpartum.[65] There was no detrimental effect on the infant/toddler responses to DTaP.[44] In a baboon model, maternal vaccination during pregnancy using an acellular vaccine prevented severe pertussis in exposed infants compared with exposed infants of unvaccinated mothers.[66] Because antipertussis antibodies are short lived, vaccination during one pregnancy may not protect the newborn in subsequent pregnancies. In 2012, the CDC recommended Tdap for pregnant women during each pregnancy.[63] Despite compelling evidence of safety and antibody transfer, uptake of Tdap vaccination during each pregnancy has been slow. A study in Michigan found 14.3% of pregnant patients on Medicaid received Tdap during pregnancy from 2011 to 2013.[67] During a pertussis outbreak in Dallas in 2012, 79% of the 220 cases occurred in infants younger than 3 months and no mother had been vaccinated during pregnancy, and only one-half had received Tdap postpartum.[68] Financial and implementation barriers must be overcome to realize achievable elimination of pertussis mortality.[69] England has had much higher success rates with the implementation of maternal Tdap vaccination, and 2 recent studies found vaccination to be safe and effective, with protection from 90% to 93% in infants younger than 2 months.[70,71] A US study using a cohort model concluded that giving Tdap during pregnancy compared with postpartum vaccination or cocooning would avoid more overall pertussis cases, hospitalizations, and deaths in addition to being more cost-effective.[72]

Multiple avenues of research are underway to improve acellular vaccines, including replacing chemically detoxified pertussis toxin with a genetically detoxified product, altering protein antigens and using adjuvants that elicit T_H1 as well as T_H2 immune responses.[4,9]

REFERENCES

1. Mooi FR. *Bordetella pertussis* and vaccination: the persistence of a genetically monomorphic pathogen. Infect Genet Evol 2010;10:36–49.
2. Clark TA. Changing pertussis epidemiology: everything old is new again. J Infect Dis 2014;209:978–81.
3. Clark TA, Messonnier NE, Hadler SC. Pertussis control: time for something new? Trends Microbiol 2012;20:211–3.
4. Plotkin SA. The pertussis problem. Clin Infect Dis 2014;58:830–3.
5. Mooi FR, Zeddeman A, van Gent M. The pertussis problem: classical epidemiology and strain characterization should go hand in hand. J Pediatr (Rio J) 2015. [Epub ahead of print].
6. Long SS, Edwards KM, Mertsola J. *Bordetella pertussis* (Pertussis) and other *Bordetella* species. In: Long SS, Pickering LK, Prober CG, editors. Princples and practice of pediatric infectious diseases. 4th edition. Edinburg (TX): Elsevier Saunders; 2012. p. 865–73.
7. Healy CM, Rench MA, Wootton SH, et al. Evaluation of the impact of a pertussis cocooning program on infant pertussis infection. Pediatr Infect Dis J 2015;34: 22–6.
8. Quinn HE, Snelling TL, Habig A, et al. Parental Tdap boosters and infant pertussis: a case-control study. Pediatrics 2014;134:713–20.
9. Mooi FR, Van Der Maas NA, De Melker HE. Pertussis resurgence: waning immunity and pathogen adaptation - two sides of the same coin. Epidemiol Infect 2014; 142:685–94.
10. Hewlett EL, Burns DL, Cotter PA, et al. Pertussis pathogenesis–what we know and what we don't know. J Infect Dis 2014;209:982–5.
11. Martin SW, Pawloski L, Williams M, et al. Pertactin-negative *Bordetella pertussis* strains: evidence for a possible selective advantage. Clin Infect Dis 2015;60: 223–7.
12. Inatsuka CS, Xu Q, Vujkovic-Cvijin I, et al. Pertactin is required for *Bordetella* species to resist neutrophil-mediated clearance. Infect Immun 2010;78:2901–9.
13. Cherry JD. Historical review of pertussis and the classical vaccine. J Infect Dis 1996;174(Suppl 3):S259–63.
14. Black RE, Cousens S, Johnson HL, et al. Global, regional, and national causes of child mortality in 2008: a systematic analysis. Lancet 2010;375:1969–87.
15. Chan MH, Ma L, Sidelinger D, et al. The California pertussis epidemic 2010: a review of 986 pediatric case reports from San Diego County. J Pediatric Infect Dis Soc 2012;1:47–54.
16. Cherry JD. Epidemic pertussis in 2012–the resurgence of a vaccine-preventable disease. N Engl J Med 2012;367:785–7.
17. Cherry JD. Pertussis in the preantibiotic and prevaccine era, with emphasis on adult pertussis. Clin Infect Dis 1999;28(Suppl 2):S107–11.
18. Winter K, Harriman K, Zipprich J, et al. California pertussis epidemic, 2010. J Pediatr 2012;161:1091–6.

19. Clark TA. Responding to pertussis. J Pediatr 2012;161:980–2.
20. Harrison CJ. Pertussis persists. Pediatric News. Available at: http://www.pediatricnews.com. Accessed January 23, 2015.
21. Centers for Disease Control and Prevention. Pertussis vaccination: acellular pertussis vaccine for reinforcing and booster use–supplementary ACIP statement. Recommendations of the Immunization Practices Advisory Committee (ACIP). MMWR Recomm Rep 1992;41(RR-1):1–10.
22. Koepke R, Eickhoff JC, Ayele RA, et al. Estimating the effectiveness of tetanus-diphtheria-acellular pertussis vaccine (Tdap) for preventing pertussis: evidence of rapidly waning immunity and difference in effectiveness by Tdap brand. J Infect Dis 2014;210:942–53.
23. Broder KR, Cortese MM, Iskander JK, et al. Preventing tetanus, diphtheria, and pertussis among adolescents: use of tetanus toxoid, reduced diphtheria toxoid and acellular pertussis vaccines recommendations of the Advisory Committee on Immunization Practices (ACIP). MMWR Recomm Rep 2006;55(RR-3):1–34.
24. Tartof SY, Lewis M, Kenyon C, et al. Waning immunity to pertussis following 5 doses of DTaP. Pediatrics 2013;131:e1047–52.
25. Misegades LK, Winter K, Harriman K, et al. Association of childhood pertussis with receipt of 5 doses of pertussis vaccine by time since last vaccine dose, California, 2010. JAMA 2012;308:2126–32.
26. Centers for Disease Control and Prevention (CDC). Pertussis epidemic–Washington, 2012. MMWR Morb Mortal Wkly Rep 2012;61:517–22.
27. Winter K, Glaser C, Watt J, et al. Pertussis epidemic–California, 2014. MMWR Morb Mortal Wkly Rep 2014;63:1129–32.
28. McGirr A, Fisman DN. Duration of pertussis immunity after DTaP immunization: a meta-analysis. Pediatrics 2015;135:331–43.
29. Klein NP, Bartlett J, Rowhani-Rahbar A, et al. Waning protection after fifth dose of acellular pertussis vaccine in children. N Engl J Med 2012;367:1012–9.
30. Witt MA, Katz PH, Witt DJ. Unexpectedly limited durability of immunity following acellular pertussis vaccination in preadolescents in a North American outbreak. Clin Infect Dis 2012;54:1730–5.
31. Witt MA, Arias L, Katz PH, et al. Reduced risk of pertussis among persons ever vaccinated with whole cell pertussis vaccine compared to recipients of acellular pertussis vaccines in a large US cohort. Clin Infect Dis 2013;56:1248–54.
32. van Gent M, Heuvelman CJ, van der heide HG, et al. Analysis of *Bordetella pertussis* clinical isolates circulating in European countries during the period 1998-2012. Eur J Clin Microbiol Infect Dis 2015;34:821–30.
33. Smallridge WE, Rolin OY, Jacobs NT, et al. Different effects of whole-cell and acellular vaccines on *Bordetella* transmission. J Infect Dis 2014;209:1981–8.
34. Hegerle N, Dore G, Guiso N. Pertactin deficient *Bordetella pertussis* present a better fitness in mice immunized with an acellular pertussis vaccine. Vaccine 2014;32:6597–600.
35. Pawloski LC, Queenan AM, Cassiday PK, et al. Prevalence and molecular characterization of pertactin-deficient *Bordetella pertussis* in the United States. Clin Vaccine Immunol 2014;21:119–25.
36. Schmidtke AJ, Boney KO, Martin SW, et al. Population diversity among *Bordetella pertussis* isolates, United States, 1935-2009. Emerg Infect Dis 2012;18:1248–55.
37. Bowden KE, Williams MM, Cassiday PK, et al. Molecular epidemiology of the pertussis epidemic in Washington State in 2012. J Clin Microbiol 2014;52:3549–57.

38. Mooi FR, van Loo IH, van Gent M, et al. *Bordetella pertussis* strains with increased toxin production associated with pertussis resurgence. Emerg Infect Dis 2009;15:1206–13.
39. Jongerius I, Schuijt TJ, Mooi FR, et al. Complement evasion by *Bordetella pertussis*: implications for improving current vaccines. J Mol Med (Berl) 2015; 93:395–402.
40. Queenan AM, Cassiday PK, Evangelista A. Pertactin-negative variants of *Bordetella pertussis* in the United States. N Engl J Med 2013;368:583–4.
41. Vodzak J, Souder E, Queenan AM, et al. In: Abstracts of the Pediatric Academic Societies Annual Meeting. Vancouver (British Columbia), May 3–6, 2014.
42. Lam C, Octavia S, Ricafort L, et al. Rapid increase in pertactin-deficient *Bordetella pertussis* isolates, Australia. Emerg Infect Dis 2014;20:626–33.
43. Tiwari T, Murphy TV, Moran J, National Immunization Program, CDC. Recommended antimicrobial agents for the treatment and postexposure prophylaxis of pertussis: 2005 CDC Guidelines. MMWR Recomm Rep 2005; 54(RR-14):1–16.
44. Munoz FM, Bond NH, Maccato M, et al. Safety and immunogenicity of tetanus diphtheria and acellular pertussis (Tdap) immunization during pregnancy in mothers and infants: a randomized clinical trial. JAMA 2014;311:1760–9.
45. Marshall H, Clarke M, Rasiah K, et al. Predictors of disease severity in children hospitalized for pertussis during an epidemic. Pediatr Infect Dis J 2015;34:339–45.
46. Liu BC, McIntyre P, Kaldor J, et al. Pertussis in older adults: prospective study of risk factors and morbidity. Clin Infect Dis 2012;55:1450–6.
47. Bodilis H, Guiso N. Virulence of pertactin-negative *Bordetella pertussis* isolates from infants, France. Emerg Infect Dis 2013;19:471–4.
48. Tatti KM, Martin S, Boney KO, et al. Qualitative assessment of pertussis diagnostics in United States laboratories. Pediatr Infect Dis J 2013;32:942–5.
49. Williams MM, Taylor TH, Warshauer DM, et al. Harmonization of *Bordetella pertussis* real-time PCR diagnostics in the United States in 2012. J Clin Microbiol 2015;53:118–23.
50. Vestrheim DF, Steinbakk M, Bjornstad ML, et al. Recovery of *Bordetella pertussis* from PCR-positive nasopharyngeal samples is dependent on bacterial load. J Clin Microbiol 2012;50:4114–5.
51. Stone BL, Daly J, Srivastava R. Duration of *Bordetella pertussis* polymerase chain reaction positivity in confirmed pertussis illness. J Pediatric Infect Dis Soc 2014;3: 347–9.
52. Zeddeman A, Witteveen S, Bart MJ, et al. Studying *Bordetella pertussis* populations by use of SNPeX, a simple high-throughput single nucleotide polymorphism typing method. J Clin Microbiol 2015;53:838–46.
53. Honein MA, Paulozzi LJ, Himelright IM, et al. Infantile hypertrophic pyloric stenosis after pertussis prophylaxis with erythromcyin: a case review and cohort study. Lancet 1999;354:2101–5.
54. Cooper WO, Griffin MR, Arbogast P, et al. Very early exposure to erythromycin and infantile hypertrophic pyloric stenosis. Arch Pediatr Adolesc Med 2002; 156:647–50.
55. Eberly MD, Eide MB, Thompson JL, et al. Azithromycin in early infancy and pyloric stenosis. Pediatrics 2015;135:483–8.
56. Munoz FM. Pertussis in infants, children, and adolescents: diagnosis, treatment, and prevention. Semin Pediatr Infect Dis 2006;17:14–9.
57. Kuperman A, Hoffmann Y, Glikman D, et al. Severe pertussis and hyperleukocytosis: is it time to change for exchange? Transfusion 2014;54:1630–3.

58. Centers for Disease Control and Prevention. Epidemiology and prevention of vaccine-preventable diseases. In: Hamborsky J, Kroger A, Wolfe C, editors. 13th edition. Washington, DC: Public Health Foundation; 2015. p. 261–76.
59. Barlow RS, Reynolds LE, Cieslak PR, et al. Vaccinated children and adolescents with pertussis infections experience reduced illness severity and duration, Oregon, 2010-2012. Clin Infect Dis 2014;58:1523–9.
60. Tiwari TS, Baughman AL, Clark TA. First pertussis vaccine dose and prevention of infant mortality. Pediatrics 2015;135:990–9.
61. Castagnini LA, Healy CM, Rench MA, et al. Impact of maternal postpartum tetanus and diphtheria toxoids and acellular pertussis immunization on infant pertussis infection. Clin Infect Dis 2012;54:78–84.
62. ACOG Committee Opinion No. 566: update on immunization and pregnancy: tetanus, diphtheria, and pertussis vaccination. Obstet Gynecol 2013;121:1411–4.
63. Centers for Disease Control and Prevention. Updated recommendations for use of tetanus toxoid, reduced diphtheria toxoid, and acellular pertussis vaccine (Tdap) in pregnant women–Advisory Committee on Immunization Practices (ACIP), 2012. MMWR Morb Mortal Wkly Rep 2013;62:131–5.
64. Chu HY, Englund JA. Maternal immunization. Clin Infect Dis 2014;59:560–8.
65. Shakib JH, Korgenski K, Sheng X, et al. Tetanus, diphtheria, acellular pertussis vaccine during pregnancy: pregnancy and infant health outcomes. J Pediatr 2013;163:1422–6.e1–4.
66. Warfel JM, Papin JF, Wolf RF, et al. Maternal and neonatal vaccination protects newborn baboons from pertussis infection. J Infect Dis 2014;210:604–10.
67. Housey M, Zhang F, Miller C, et al. Vaccination with tetanus, diphtheria, and acellular pertussis vaccine of pregnant women enrolled in Medicaid–Michigan, 2011-2013. MMWR Morb Mortal Wkly Rep 2014;63:839–42.
68. Cantey JB, Sanchez PJ, Tran J, et al. Pertussis: a persistent cause of morbidity and mortality in young infants. J Pediatr 2014;164:1489–92.e1.
69. Cherry JD. Tetanus-diphtheria-pertussis immunization in pregnant women and the prevention of pertussis in young infants. Clin Infect Dis 2015;60:338–40.
70. Amirthalingam G, Andrews N, Campbell H, et al. Effectiveness of maternal pertussis vaccination in England: an observational study. Lancet 2014;384:1521–8.
71. Dabrera G, Amirthalingam G, Andrews N, et al. A case-control study to estimate the effectiveness of maternal pertussis vaccination in protecting newborn infants in England and Wales, 2012-2013. Clin Infect Dis 2015;60:333–7.
72. Terranella A, Asay GR, Messonnier ML, et al. Pregnancy dose Tdap and postpartum cocooning to prevent infant pertussis: a decision analysis. Pediatrics 2013;131:e1748–56.

The Expanded Impact of Human Papillomavirus Vaccine

Barbara A. Pahud, MD, MPH[a],*, Kevin A. Ault, MD[b]

KEYWORDS

- Human papilloma virus • Vaccine • Cancer • Adolescent • Immunization programs
- Health promotion

KEY POINTS

- HPV is the most common sexually transmitted infection in the US and in the world. Almost all females and males will be infected with at least one type of HPV at some point in their lives.
- Some HPV virus types have oncogenic potential resulting in various types of anogenital, head and neck cancers in both males and females.
- HPV is responsible for essentially all cervical cancer among women and has become the most common cause of oropharyngeal cancers.
- Despite ongoing efforts from providers and established guidelines, national coverage with the recommended three doses of HPV vaccine is inadequate.
- The HPV vaccine has been shown to be both safe and efficacious in preventing life-threatening sexually transmitted cancers as well as genital and non-genital warts.

INTRODUCTION

Human papilloma virus (HPV) infection is the most common sexually transmitted infection (STI) infection in the United States. Most infections are asymptomatic and transient, but some infections will result in anogenital warts and anogenital or oropharyngeal cancers in both men and women. Because of the large proportion of people exposed, preventing HPV infection is a public health priority to reduce cancer and HPV-associated complications. Because screening is only available for cervical cancer, and there is a significant cost to HPV-associated disease, prevention though vaccination is the most cost-effective and lifesaving intervention currently available

[a] Division of Infectious Diseases, Department of Pediatrics, Children's Mercy Hospital, University of Missouri, Kansas City (UMKC), 2401 Gillham Road, Kansas City, MO 64108, USA; [b] Department of Obstetrics and Gynecology, University of Kansas Medical Center, 3901 Rainbow Boulevard, Kansas City, KS 66160, USA
* Corresponding author.
E-mail address: bapahud@cmh.edu

Infect Dis Clin N Am 29 (2015) 715–724
http://dx.doi.org/10.1016/j.idc.2015.07.007
0891-5520/15/$ – see front matter © 2015 Elsevier Inc. All rights reserved.

id.theclinics.com

to decrease the burden of HPV-related cancers and other HPV-associated diseases. It is critical for pediatricians to regard HPV vaccination as a cancer-preventing intervention and to make a strong recommendation for early and timely vaccination and completion of the 3-dose series. The goal of early vaccination is to immunize prior to first exposure to HPV virus; thus early vaccination is critical to ensure cancer prevention. Prevention is cheap compared with the cost of cancer and its complications, including premature birth, infertility, and even death.

ETIOLOGY

HPV is a double-stranded circular nonenveloped DNA virus of the Papillomaviridae family. HPVs encode 2 structural proteins (L) in a circular genome enclosed in a capsid shell. The major capsid protein L1 encodes for monomers that spontaneously self-assemble to form pentamers that can then form empty shells that resemble a virus, known as virus-like particles (VLPs). The minor capsid protein L2 has functions required for host infection.

Other genes in the circular genome are responsible for transcription, replication, and interacting with the host; some of these have oncogenic potential due to their ability to modulate the activity of p53 and other cell cycle's regulation processes and block apoptosis.[1] There are more than 150 HPV genotypes (types) or strains. Genital HPV types are categorized as high-risk types or low-risk types based on their association with cervical cancer. The most prevalent high-risk types in the United States are types 16 and 18. They cause high-grade cervical cell abnormalities that are precursors to cancer. Low-risk types such as types 6 and 11 do not contribute to the incidence of high-grade dysplasia (precancerous lesions) or cervical cancer, but can cause benign or low-grade cervical cell changes, resulting in genital warts and respiratory or laryngeal papillomatosis.

INCIDENCE AND PREVALENCE

HPV is the most common STI in the United States and in the world.[2] Nearly every American will be infected with at least 1 type of HPV at some point in their lives. The estimated risk of acquiring an HPV infection in men is 70% to 98 % and 54% to 95 %, for women.[3]

There are currently an estimated 79 million Americans infected with 14 million new infections per year. The 2 most prevalent types are HPV16 and HPV18, likely reflecting their evolutionary advantage due to their oncogenic potential. These 2 types are responsible for over 60% of all invasive HPV-associated cancers in the United States (approximately 21,300 cases annually).[4]

TRANSMISSION

HPV is highly transmissible, with peak incidence soon after the onset of sexual activity.[5] It is transmitted through skin-to-skin contact (noncoital behaviors) and through vaginal, anal, or oral intercourse. It is important to note that intercourse is not necessary to become infected.

Because HPV can infect skin that is not covered by a condom, condoms do not completely stop transmission of HPV, but lower prevalence has been reported among consistent condom users.[6]

HPV may be transmitted more often from women to men than from men to women.[7] HPV infection risk is associated with the number of lifetime sex partners for both men and women.[8]

CLINICAL PRESENTATION
Asymptomatic

Most people never know that they have been infected unless a woman has an abnormal pap test with a positive HPV test. More than 90% of detected infections are cleared within 2 years of acquisition. About 10% of infections will not clear on their own and will thus result in HPV-related disease in the form of genital warts, dysplasia, or cancer.

Warts

Also referred to as condylomata acuminata, or venereal warts, HPV 6 and HPV 11 are responsible for over 90% of all genital warts. Coinfection with other types is possible, combining both low- and high risk lesions. Low-risk HPV infections carry significant morbidity because of psychosocial and economic burden, due to stigma associated with the disease and fear of cancer. Approximately 1% of sexually active young adults have genital warts. Lifetime rates of genital warts have been estimated at 4% to 7 % in a study done in the United States.[9] Prevalence rates are highest in women and men in their twenties and early thirties.

Cancer

HPV infection has been identified as a human carcinogen for 6 types of cancers, including cervix, penis, vulva, vagina, anus, and oropharynx. Cervical cancer is the most preventable of all of the female cancers. However, even with an excellent cervical cancer screening program in the United States, there are still around 12,000 case of cervical cancer each year in this country and 4000 attributable deaths in 2011.[10] In addition to invasive cancers, it is estimated that there are 1.4 million cervical disease or preinvasive cervical cancers and another 40,000 of the highest grade of anal, vulvar and vaginal precancers. Rates of HPV-related anal and oropharyngeal cancers are increasing. **Fig. 1** shows the estimated number of HPV-related cancers in the United States. Among males, the most common HPV related cancer was oropharyngeal cancer. More oropharyngeal cancers that were previously thought to be caused by tobacco and/or alcohol use are now being identified as HPV-related cancers. The number of oropharyngeal cancers diagnosed that are not caused by HPV have declined by half, likely because of decreased use of tobacco and alcohol, but prevalence of oropharyngeal cancers increased from 16% (1984–1989) to 72% (2000–2004), mostly due to HPV-16.[11] Patients with HPV-positive oropharyngeal cancer are more likely to be young, male, and white, but also HPV associated-oropharyngeal cancers have better survival. At this

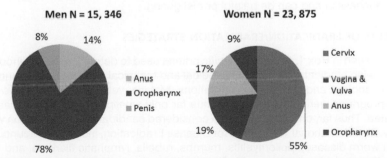

Fig. 1. Estimated HPV-related cancers United States, 2015. (*Data from* Saraiya M, Unger ER, Thompson TD, et al. US assessment of HPV types in cancers: implications for current and 9-Valent HPV vaccines. J Natl Cancer Inst 2015;107(6):djv086.)

rate, HPV-related oropharyngeal cancers may exceed the cervical cancers by the year 2020.[12] There is no pap test equivalent to screen for oropharyngeal cancers; thus primary prevention with vaccination should be emphasized in both men and women.

Special Populations

Some subpopulations are at increased risk for HPV-related diseases, including cancer. Immunosuppression is the underlying cause in many of these patients. It has long been known that women with solid organ transplants are at increased risk of cervical cancer. Men and women with human immunodeficiency virus (HIV) are at increased risk of cervical and anal cancers. Men who have sex with men are also at increased risk of anal dysplasia and anal cancer.

DIAGNOSIS
Molecular Testing

Most infections are not diagnosed, as they are asymptomatic, although several tests have been approved for HPV diagnostic testing in women. This is done as part of a strategy for screening for cervical dysplasia and cervical cancer. There is no approved equivalent pap test for screening for anal or oropharyngeal cancers.

Serology

HPV avoids host immune response, because these viruses are nonlytic viruses and are restricted to the squamous and glandular epithelium, going undetected and unrecognized by the immune system. Not all infected persons develop detectable antibody, and correlates of immunity have not been established. Serum antibodies against many different viral products have been demonstrated but are mostly used for research trials. The best-characterized antibodies are those directed against conformational epitopes of the L1 capsid protein assembled as VLPs used in the currently available vaccine.

TREATMENT/COMPLICATIONS

HPV infections are treated based on their clinical manifestations. Organized screening programs will detect HPV-related cervical dysplasia. These premalignant lesions are usually treated with surgery, including cryotherapy, laser ablation, and surgical excision. Treatment for cervical dysplasia is associated with a subsequent increased risk of preterm birth. Treatment of anal dysplasia likewise involves ablation or other similar surgeries. Many treatments have been described for genital warts. None are entirely successful and can be painful or disfiguring.

PROSPECTS OF ERADICATION/ERADICATION STRATEGIES

As can be seen in **Box 1**, there are specific criteria used to determine the likelihood of a disease being eradicated based on biological and technical feasibility, costs and benefits, and societal and political considerations. Malaria, yellow fever, and yaws eradication programs were attempted, but thus far only smallpox has been successfully eradicated. Thus far, only 6 diseases are considered candidates for eradication worldwide by The International Task Force for Disease Eradication, including dracunculiasis (Guinea worm disease), poliomyelitis, mumps, rubella, lymphatic filariasis, and taeniasis/cysticercosis (pork tapeworm). Factors that may make eradication impossible today, however, may change tomorrow and allow eradication in the future. Even though a vaccine is now available against some HPV serotypes that is both safe

---

Box 1
Criteria for assessing eradicability of diseases and conditions

- Scientific Feasibility

  ○ Epidemiologic vulnerability (eg, existence of nonhuman reservoir, ease of spread, natural cyclical decline in prevalence, naturally induced immunity, ease of diagnosis, and duration of any relapse potential)

  ○ Effective, practical intervention available (eg, vaccine or other primary preventive, curative treatment, and means of eliminating vector). Ideally, intervention should be effective, safe, inexpensive, long-lasting, and easily deployed.

  ○ Demonstrated feasibility of elimination (eg, documented elimination from island or other geographic unit)

- Political Will/Popular Support

  ○ Perceived burden of the disease (eg, extent, deaths, other effects; true burden may not be perceived; the reverse of benefits expected to accrue from eradication; relevance to rich and poor countries).

  ○ Expected cost of eradication (especially in relation to perceived burden from the disease).

  ○ Synergy of eradication efforts with other interventions (eg, potential for added benefits or savings or spin-off effects)

  ○ Necessity for eradication rather than control

From Centers for Disease Control and Prevention. Recommendations of the International Task Force for Disease Eradication. MMWR 1993;42(No. RR-16):1–38.

---

and effective, the vaccine does not cover all available serotypes. In addition, there is not sufficient political will or popular support to implement universal immunization at this moment.

AVAILABLE VACCINES

HPV vaccines are made of the HPV L1 protein, the major capsid protein of HPV through recombinant DNA technology. L1 protein is expressed producing noninfectious virus-like particles (VLP) that resemble the wild-type HPV virus. VLPs are noninfectious and nononcogenic. These VLP proteins are designed to produce a virus-neutralizing antibody response to prevent initial infection by the HPV types found in each vaccine. HPV vaccines produce high levels of neutralizing antibody by eliciting a strong B-cell mediated immune response, which provides long-term immunity, better than natural infection.[13,14]

There are 2 brands of HPV vaccine on the market, Gardasil and Cervarix, with 3 products available conferring protection against 2, 4, or 9 serotypes (2vHPV, 4vHPV, and 9vHPV). Both brands target the 2 types of HPV (16, 18) that cause over 60% of all HPV-associated cancers in the United States (65% for females, 63% for males, approximately 21,300 cases annually). Both vaccine brands have been shown to prevent cervical precancers in women. Both vaccines are given as shots and require 3 doses, although on slightly different schedules (**Table 1**). Each vaccine brand uses a different adjuvant. Gardasil vaccines (4vHPV and 9vHPV) also protect against HPV types 6 and 11, the types that responsible for 90% of anogenital warts (condylomata) in women and men and most cases of recurrent respiratory papillomatosis.[15] Cervarix and Gardasil are approved for girls, while Gardasil has been tested and licensed for use in boys

Table 1
Human papilloma virus vaccines licensed for use in the United States

Vaccine	Bivalent	Quadrivalent (Expected to Fase out by Mid-2016)	Nanovalent
Brand Name (manufacturer)	Cervarix (GSK)	Gardasil (Merck)	Gardasil 9 (Merck)
Virus-like-particle serotypes	16, 18	6, 11, 16, 18	6, 11, 16, 18, 31, 33, 45, 52, 58
Doses/interval	0, 1, and 6 mo	0, 2 and 6 mo	
Manufacturing	*Trichoplusia ni* insect cell line infected with L1 encoding recombinant baculovirus	*Saccharomyces cerevisiae* (Baker's yeast), expressing L1	
Adjuvant	500 μg aluminum hydroxide, 50 μg 3-O-desacyl-4' monophosphoryl lipid A	225 μg amorphous aluminum hydroxyphosphate sulfate	500 μg amorphous aluminum hydroxyphosphate sulfate
FDA approval	Females only	Males/Females	Females 9 through 26 y Males aged 9 through 15 y

Adapted from Petrosky E, Bocchini JA Jr, Hariri S, et al. Use of 9-valent human papillomavirus (HPV) vaccine: updated HPV vaccination recommendations of the advisory committee on immunization practices. MMWR Morb Mortal Wkly Rep 2015;64(11):300–4.

also. Although both vaccine brands protect against HPV16, which is the most common HPV type responsible for HPV-associated cancers including cancers of cervix, vulva, vagina, penis, and anus and oropharynx, only Gardasil has been tested and shown to protect against precancers of the vulva, vagina, and anus.

The new 9-valent human papillomavirus vaccine (9vHPV) includes 7 cancer-causing HPV-types: 16 and 18 (already included in the bivalent and quadrivalent vaccine) plus 31, 33, 45, 52, and 58. In the United States, approximately 10% of invasive HPV-associated cancers are attributable to the 5 additional types in 9vHPV: HPV 31, 33, 45, 52, and 58 (14% for women; 4% for men, approximately 3400 cases annually). These serotypes tend to be more prevalent in minority women. In addition to the expanded protection against cervical cancer in certain minorities, the new 9-valent vaccine has the potential to protect against an additional 8% of oropharyngeal cancers, the second-most-common HPV-associated cancer.[16] The new 9-valent vaccine will eventually become the only Gardasil product, replacing completely the 4vHPV vaccine (expected to phase out by mid-2016). HPV-related cancers prevented by the new 9-valent HPV vaccine can be seen in **Fig. 2**.

Human Papilloma Virus Vaccines Advisory Committee on Immunization Practices Indications

Routine use
Routine use is recommended for all boys and girls ages 11 to 12.[2] The Advisory Committee on Immunization Practices (ACIP) recently updated its recommendations on HPV vaccine to include the new 9-valent HPV vaccine.[4] There is no preferential use for 9vHPV product over 4vHPV or 2vHPV as of June 2015, but this may change in a future ACIP vote. For girls, there is no preferential formulation, but for boys, only Gardasil products are approved.

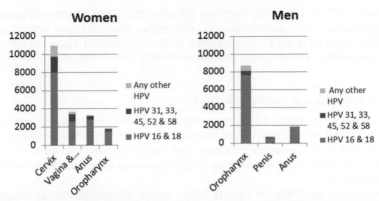

Fig. 2. HPV related cancers prevented by 9-valent vaccine, United States, 2015. (*Data from* Saraiya M, Unger ER, Thompson TD, et al. US assessment of HPV types in cancers: implications for current and 9-Valent HPV vaccines. J Natl Cancer Inst 2015;107(6):djv086.)

Catch-up ages

Catch-up ages doses are indicated for 13 to 21 years in males and 13 to 26 years in females.

Permissive use

The vaccine is approved by the US Food and Drug Administration (FDA) for ages 9 to 10; thus vaccination series may be started early.

It is also recommended for men ages 22 to 26 years, especially in men who have sex with men.

Vaccine Safety

More than 175 million doses of HPV vaccine have been distributed worldwide, and 57 million doses have been distributed in the United States since 2006. No serious safety concerns have been identified since vaccine introduction.

The most common adverse events reported were considered mild. These findings are similar to the safety reviews of the other 2 recommended teen vaccines, meningococcal vaccines and tetanus booster vaccines.

For serious adverse events reported, there has been no unusual pattern or clustering that would suggest that the events were caused by the HPV vaccine. As with all vaccines, there is continuous monitoring of the safety of these vaccines with phase 4 clinical trials and through vaccine adverse events reporting system (VAERS). These vaccine safety studies continue to show that HPV vaccines are safe.

Vaccine Efficacy

Prior to vaccine introduction, the overall prevalence of any HPV was about 40% among females aged 14 to 59 years.[15] After vaccine introduction, despite low vaccination coverage and a female-only recommendation for vaccination, National Health and Nutrition Examination Survey (NHANES) data showed that HPV prevalence for the vaccine serotypes declined by half (from 11.5% in 2003–2006 to 5.1% in 2007–2010) in 14- to 19-year-old women, the targeted age group.[17] Other age groups did not show a statistically significant difference over time. Based on these data, vaccine effectiveness for the prevention of infection was estimated at 82%.

High HPV vaccination coverage in other countries such as Australia has resulted in the added benefit of herd immunity and associated decreased risk of HPV transmission.[18,19] All 3 available vaccines are more than 90% effective at generating immune responses and seroconversion, preventing infections and lesions caused by the HPV types included in the vaccines, particularly among those not infected at time of vaccination. Efficacy has been seen in all clinical sites where HPV causes disease.

Vaccine Precautions and Contraindications

Those being vaccinated may develop syncope, which may result in falling with injury. A trend of increased reports of syncope after vaccination has been especially prevalent since introduction of adolescent vaccines. As is recommended with administration of any other adolescent vaccine, observation for 15 minutes after vaccine administration is recommended.

Vaccine is contraindicated in anyone with a severe allergic reaction or anaphylaxis to any vaccine component or a prior dose of HPV vaccine. Allergic reactions in latex-sensitive individuals may occur with administration of the 2vHPV, as the tip caps of the prefilled syringes may contain natural rubber latex. Anaphylactic reactions to latex are a contraindication to vaccination. The 4vHPV and 9VHPV contain trace amount of yeast protein and are contraindicated in allergic patients. HPV vaccination is not recommended for pregnant women.

RESEARCH NEEDS

The next generation of prophylactic HPV vaccines should aim to overcome some of the limitations of the current vaccines. Challenges and opportunities to overcome include

- Mix-and-match studies. It is important to understand if immunogenicity of HPV vaccine varies if different products are utilized.
- Need for additional 9vHPV dose when series completed. With the availability of HPV-9, the ACIP will need to make a recommendation for children who have completed the series with 2vHPV or 4vHPV. The recommendation may be to provide one or more additional doses of 9vHPV to confer protection against the additional serotypes. Currently there are no recommendations to give additional doses of 9vHPV to individuals who have completed the 3-dose series with another version of the HPV vaccine.
- Potential of single-dose protection. A single dose or reduced number of doses would increase compliance and help increase vaccination coverage in the United States. In developing countries, decreasing the number of doses required would increase access because of understandable logistical and economic reasons. Previous research has shown that 3 doses provide 90% protection against serotype 16 and 18. Post hoc analysis that was not randomized showed that those who received only 1 or 2 doses had very similar results, with 90% protection for the 2 doses, and even higher protection for 1 dose, although the single-dose group was limited by numbers with overlapping confidence intervals. The analysis adds more data to the suspicion that although 3 doses of vaccine are optimal and currently recommended in the United States, 2 doses or even 1 dose may offer substantial protection.
- Optimal spacing of doses to increase compliance and optimize immunogenicity. Research shows that women who received only 2 doses of HPV do not see any cross-protection for 31, 33, 45 unless the spacing between the 2 vaccines is 6 months apart instead of the current recommendation. The current

recommended dosing schedule does not demonstrate any added benefit, so further research into optimal priming and boosting is needed.

- Development of a generic vaccine. New vaccines targeting L2 (another minor capsid protein that is not type specific) instead of L1 to increase protection against multiple types is on the horizon. This is especially important for minorities and developing nations, which may have different prevalence of types than the United States. On a global basis, the next most prevalent types are HPV 31, 33, and 45, so the goal is to target the next more critical HPV types.
- Increase vaccination coverage. If the United States were able to increase vaccination coverage, it is known based on data from other countries that have successfully vaccinated, the United States could reach herd protection levels and have a significant impact on HPV-related diseases. Coverage in the states that have the lowest vaccination rates for HPV have the highest rates of cervical cancer and deaths from the disease (data presented at AACR- American Association for Cancer Research, University of North Carolina).[20]
- Develop strategies to help providers make a strong recommendation for HPV vaccine at the indicated age or earlier. Parents and teens who knew more about HPV were no more likely than those with less HPV knowledge to get the vaccine for themselves or their daughters.
- Evaluate impact on disease prevention when vaccine is not given on time. Half of girls receive the first dose of the vaccine after age 12.[21] It is not certain how effective the vaccine will be at protecting against HPV when the chances of infection prior to immunization are higher. Develop strategies to increase vaccination on time.

REFERENCES

1. Doorbar J, Quint W, Banks L, et al. The biology and life-cycle of human papillomaviruses. Vaccine 2012;30(Suppl 5):F55–70.
2. Markowitz LE, Dunne EF, Saraiya M, et al. Human papillomavirus vaccination: recommendations of the Advisory Committee on Immunization Practices (ACIP). MMWR Recomm Rep 2014;63:1–30.
3. Chesson HW, Dunne EF, Hariri S, et al. The estimated lifetime probability of acquiring human papillomavirus in the United States. Sex Transm Dis 2014;41:660–4.
4. Petrosky E, Bocchini JA Jr, Hariri S, et al. Use of 9-Valent Human Papillomavirus (HPV) Vaccine: Updated HPV vaccination recommendations of the advisory committee on immunization practices. MMWR Morb Mortal Wkly Rep 2015;64:300–4.
5. Munoz N, Mendez F, Posso H, et al. Incidence, duration, and determinants of cervical human papillomavirus infection in a cohort of Colombian women with normal cytological results. J Infect Dis 2004;190:2077–87.
6. Winer RL, Hughes JP, Feng Q, et al. Condom use and the risk of genital human papillomavirus infection in young women. N Engl J Med 2006;354:2645–54.
7. Nyitray AG, Lin H-Y, Fulp WJ, et al. The role of monogamy and duration of heterosexual relationships in human papillomavirus transmission. J Infect Dis 2014;209:1007–15.
8. Vaccarella S, Franceschi S, Herrero R, et al. Sexual behavior, condom use, and human papillomavirus: pooled analysis of the IARC human papillomavirus prevalence surveys. Cancer Epidemiol Biomarkers Prev 2006;15:326–33.
9. Patel H, Wagner M, Singhal P, et al. Systematic review of the incidence and prevalence of genital warts. BMC Infect Dis 2013;13:39.

10. Group USCSW. United States Cancer Statistics: 1999–2011 incidence and Mortality Web-based report. Atlanta (GA): U.S. Department of Health and Human Services, Centers for Disease Control and Prevention and National Cancer Institute; 2014.
11. Chaturvedi AK, Engels EA, Pfeiffer RM, et al. Human papillomavirus and rising oropharyngeal cancer incidence in the United States. J Clin Oncol 2011;29: 4294–301.
12. Kreimer AR, Chaturvedi AK. HPV-associated oropharyngeal cancers—are they preventable? Cancer Prev Res (Phila) 2011;4:1346–9.
13. Roteli-Martins CM, Naud P, De Borba P, et al. Sustained immunogenicity and efficacy of the HPV-16/18 AS04-adjuvanted vaccine: up to 8.4 years of follow-up. Hum Vaccine Immunother 2012;8:390–7.
14. Nygard M, Saah A, Munk C, et al. Evaluation of the long-term anti-HPV 6, 11, 16, and 18 immune responses generated by gardasil®. Clin Vaccine Immunol 2015; 22(8):943–8.
15. Hariri S, Unger ER, Sternberg M, et al. Prevalence of genital human papillomavirus among females in the United States, the National Health And Nutrition Examination Survey, 2003-2006. J Infect Dis 2011;204:566–73.
16. Saraiya M, Unger ER, Thompson TD, et al. US assessment of HPV Types in cancers: implications for current and 9-valent HPV vaccines. J Natl Cancer Inst 2015; 107:djv086.
17. Markowitz LE, Hariri S, Lin C, et al. Reduction in human papillomavirus (HPV) prevalence among young women following HPV vaccine introduction in the United States, National Health and Nutrition Examination Surveys, 2003-2010. J Infect Dis 2013;208:385–93.
18. Donovan B, Franklin N, Guy R, et al. Quadrivalent human papillomavirus vaccination and trends in genital warts in Australia: analysis of national sentinel surveillance data. Lancet Infect Dis 2011;11:39–44.
19. Smith MA, Lew JB, Walker RJ, et al. The predicted impact of HPV vaccination on male infections and male HPV-related cancers in Australia. Vaccine 2011;29: 9112–22.
20. Brewer N. In search of racial disparities in HPV vaccination. Poster presented at AACR Meeting. November 9, 2014.
21. Rahman M, McGrath CJ, Hirth JM, et al. Age at HPV vaccine initiation and completion among US adolescent girls: trend from 2008 to 2012. Vaccine 2015;33:585–7.

Measles 50 Years After Use of Measles Vaccine

James L. Goodson, BSN, MPH[a],*, Jane F. Seward, MBBS, MPH[b]

KEYWORDS

- Measles elimination • Vaccine preventable • Vaccination • Exemptions • Mortality
- Rash • Fever

KEY POINTS

- Measles can be severe; globally, measles causes an estimated 400 deaths each day.
- Measles still occurs in the United States following virus importations, primarily among intentionally unvaccinated children and young adults; clinicians should keep measles in their differential diagnosis of febrile rash illness and encourage on-time, complete vaccinations.
- Measles can and should be eradicated, and all 6 World Health Organization (WHO) regions have set a goal for measles elimination by or before 2020; continued global funding and support are key strategies to achieve these goals.
- Until measles is eliminated globally, public health agencies will need to remain vigilant and on the frontline to maintain measles outbreak preparedness and rapid response capacity to contain outbreaks when they occur.

INTRODUCTION

Before the availability of measles vaccine in 1963, measles was a common childhood disease that caused an estimated 135 million cases of measles and more than 6 million measles-related deaths globally each year, including an estimated 4 million cases and 450 deaths in the United States.[1-3] Although measles was eliminated from the United States in 2000, measles still occurs following measles virus importations from other countries, most commonly by unvaccinated US residents who become infected while traveling abroad. These importations can result in measles outbreaks if the measles-infected

The authors have nothing to disclose. The findings and conclusions in this report are those of the authors and do not necessarily represent the official position of the CDC.
[a] Global Immunization Division, Center for Global Health, Centers for Disease Control and Prevention, 1600 Clifton Road, Northeast, MS A-04, Atlanta, GA 30333, USA; [b] Division of Viral Diseases, National Center for Immunization and Respiratory Diseases, Centers for Disease Control and Prevention, 1600 Clifton Road, Northeast, Atlanta, GA 30333, USA
* Corresponding author.
E-mail address: jgoodson@cdc.gov

Infect Dis Clin N Am 29 (2015) 725–743
http://dx.doi.org/10.1016/j.idc.2015.08.001
0891-5520/15/$ – see front matter Published by Elsevier Inc.

id.theclinics.com

person comes in contact with susceptible persons, particularly in communities with low vaccination coverage. In recent years, the annual number of reported measles cases in the United States has increased and larger outbreaks have occurred, predominantly among persons who are unvaccinated by choice.[4] Today, many physicians are less familiar with the clinical presentation of measles and do not always keep measles in mind for the differential diagnosis of febrile rash illness. This article reviews experience with a half century of use of measles vaccine in the United States and globally, including the historical perspective of the virus, events leading to vaccine development, vaccine safety, effectiveness and impact, clinical manifestations, and the current challenges and future considerations for measles eradication.

MEASLES HISTORICAL ASPECTS AND VIROLOGY

Measles virus emerged more than 1000 years ago when our human ancestors domesticated cattle.[5,6] Close contact with domesticated cattle over a prolonged period likely allowed the animal virus rinderpest to mutate enough to make the transition from cows to humans as host. Humans are the only natural host for sustaining measles virus transmission. Clinical measles was first described and differentiated from smallpox in the tenth century by the Persian physician Rhazes. After emerging as an Old World virus, measles became endemic in humans; after importations into the Western Hemisphere from trans-Atlantic human migration, measles caused massive devastation, disease, and death among entirely measles-susceptible populations in the New World.[7] Measles was first described in the United States in Boston in 1657 and became endemic, causing periodic severe epidemics resulting in substantial illness and death.[5,6]

Measles virus was first isolated from a measles-infected boy (Edmonston-B strain) in the United States by Thomas C. Peebles while he was working in the Children's Hospital Boston laboratory of John F. Enders in 1954 (**Fig. 1**).[8] The virus is a negative-strand RNA virus that belongs to the genus *Morbillivirus* of the family Paramyxoviridae. Measles virus is monotypic with only one serotype. The full genomes of vaccine and wild-type strains have been sequenced.[9] The WHO Global Measles and Rubella Laboratory Network established a set of reference sequences for these genotypes and periodically updates measles virus nomenclature; WHO recognizes 24 measles virus genotypes, organized into 8 clades of measles (A–H).[10]

MEASLES PATHOGENESIS

The pathogenesis of measles is not fully understood; however, the development of new molecular techniques has recently advanced pathogenesis studies. The initial measles virus infection occurs via cell entry of measles virus into the respiratory tract, although the cell receptors and specific target cells are not well defined. From the respiratory tract, the virus enters the lymphatic system where virus amplification occurs, leading to acute viremia. In the blood, monocytes and lymphocytes become infected and carry the virus to organs throughout the body.[11,12] Measles virus enters and replicates in the lymphoid tissues and organs, including the skin, lungs, gastrointestinal tract, liver, and kidneys.[13] Measles virus infection of white blood cells leads to a decline in CD4 lymphocytes and causes transient immunosuppression starting before the rash and lasting up to at least 1 month; however, the duration and specific mechanisms leading to immune system dysregulation are unknown. Measles infection induces robust humoral and cellular immune responses, resulting in lifelong immunity.

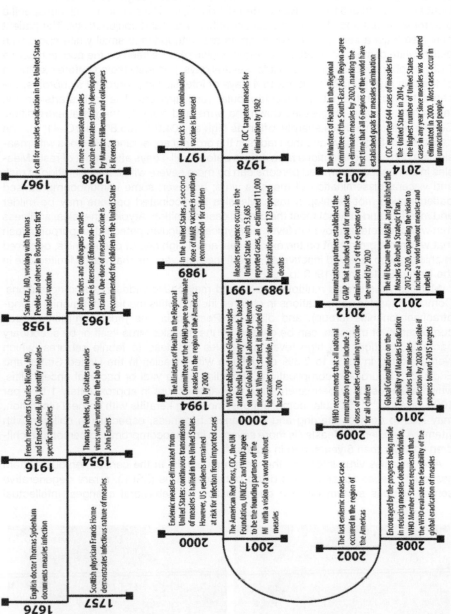

Fig. 1. Historical events on the path to a world without measles. CDC, Centers for Disease Control and Prevention; GVAP, Global Vaccine Action Plan; M&RI, Measles & Rubella Initiative; MI, Measles Initiative; MMR, measles-mumps-rubella; PAHO, Pan American Health Organization; UN, United Nations; UNICEF, United Nation Children's Fund.

DISEASE DESCRIPTION

Measles is a highly contagious virus that spreads through the air via droplets and aerosolized respiratory secretions when an infected person coughs or sneezes. After an incubation period of 8 to 12 days (range 7–21 days), the illness begins with nonspecific prodromal symptoms of fever, malaise, cough, coryza, and conjunctivitis. The patient may also have a sore throat. Koplik spots are pathognomic small white spots with bluish-white centers on a red background, which may be seen on the buccal mucosa 1 day before rash onset and persist for several days, generally fading before resolution of the skin rash (**Fig. 2**).[14] After 2 to 4 days of intensifying prodromal symptoms, the characteristic erythematous maculopapular rash appears. The rash starts on the face and neck and progresses down the arms and trunk to the distal extremities. Concurrently, fever rises sharply, often as high as 104.0°F 105.8°F (40°C–41°C). The rash lasts for 3 to 7 days and then fades in the order of appearance. Persons with measles are considered infectious from 4 days before until 4 days after onset of rash. Measles in immunocompromised persons can be more severe with longer duration of rash and visceral dissemination of measles virus; however, some immunocompromised patients might not develop a rash. Measles in vaccinated persons may be milder and modified and may not meet the clinical case definition. Atypical measles, an illness that was characterized by high fever, an atypical (vesicular, petechial, or purpuric) rash that was most prominent on the extremities, and a high rate of pneumonitis, occurred in children who received inactivated (killed) measles vaccine that was in limited use in the United States from 1963 to 1968.[15,16]

Measles virus infects multiple organs and may cause widespread complications. Common measles complications in children include otitis media, pneumonia, laryngotracheobronchitis (croup), and diarrhea. Pneumonia, the most common serious complication of measles, can be caused by the measles virus itself or by secondary bacterial infection. The high fever in measles may lead to febrile seizures, which were reported in 0.1% to 2.3% of children with measles in the United States and England.[14] Neurologic complications, including acute viral or bacterial encephalitis, which often results in permanent brain damage, occurs in approximately 1 to 4 per 1000 cases.[3,14,17,18] Ocular complications, including keratitis with corneal ulceration, may lead to corneal scarring and permanent blindness, especially in children with vitamin A deficiency. Measles is more severe in immunocompromised persons, in children younger than 5 years, and in adults.[14]

After measles virus infection, the virus may persist in the central nervous system tissue and cause subacute sclerosing panencephalitis (SSPE), a rare degenerative central nervous system disease characterized by behavioral changes, intellectual

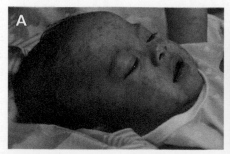 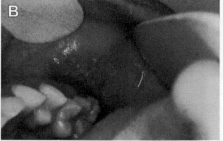

Fig. 2. Koplik spots of measles in a 7-year-old white boy. (*A*) Measles rash in infant. (*B*) Measles Koplik spots on buccal mucosa. (*Courtesy of* [*B*] Larry Frenkel, MD; with permission.)

deterioration, seizures, and death. The onset of SSPE after measles infection generally starts 6 to 10 years after the primary infection,[19] complicating its diagnosis and laboratory confirmation, particularly in limited resource settings. The global burden of SSPE is unknown, and current estimates of occurrence range from 1 in 2500 measles cases to 1 in 10,000 measles cases.[20,21] The risk for SSPE is higher when the primary measles infection occurs at a younger age.[18,22]

Poor pregnancy outcomes, including preterm birth, low birth weight, and maternal death, are associated with measles infection during pregnancy, because physiologic adaptations in the immune system during pregnancy can increase a woman's susceptibility.[23,24] Pregnant women infected with measles are more likely to be hospitalized, develop pneumonia, and die than nonpregnant women.[25,26] Previously published case series reports describe spontaneous abortion after measles infections during pregnancy; however, no studies have demonstrated unequivocally that gestational measles causes a higher rate of spontaneous abortion.[24]

PREVACCINE MEASLES DISEASE BURDEN

Before licensure and widespread use of measles vaccine through the global Expanded Program on Immunization established in 1974, measles epidemic cycles occurred every 2 to 3 years and virtually everyone experienced measles illness during childhood; more than 90% of individuals were infected by the age of 10 to 15 years.[27–29] In 1980, before widespread implementation of measles vaccine programs, measles was still estimated to cause more than 2 million deaths and between 15,000 and 60,000 cases of blindness each year in the prevaccine era.[1,30,31]

Measles became a reportable disease in the United States in 1912, and over the next decade, an average of 297,216 cases (reported measles incidence of 289 per 100,000 population) and 5948 measles-related deaths were reported each year, primarily among children younger than 5 years.[32] Over subsequent decades, measles deaths declined as sanitation and medical care improved; nevertheless, in the immediate prevaccine era (1956-1960), an estimated 4 million measles cases occurred every year in the United States, which resulted in an estimated 48,000 hospitalizations and an average of 450 reported deaths.[33] Reporting of measles cases was only 10% to 15% complete; the average annual number of reported measles cases during 1956-1960 was 530,217 and the reported measles incidence was 310 cases per 100,000 population.[32,34] In the immediate prevaccine era, serologic studies indicated that the highest age-specific incidence was in children aged 3 to 6 years and the highest case fatality rates were in very young children, younger than 2 years.[29]

MEASLES EPIDEMIOLOGY

In the United States, following the recommendation for routine use of measles vaccine for children aged 9 months—the initial age recommended for vaccination—measles cases declined 60% by 1966 (**Fig. 3**).[32] In 1967, a call was made for measles eradication in the United States.[35] From 1967 until 2000, 3 initiatives for measles elimination were launched. The 1967 initiative advocated 4 strategies: (1) routine vaccination of infants, (2) vaccination of all susceptible children at school entry, (3) surveillance, and (4) epidemic control.[32] Initial successes with reported measles cases declining 95% by 1968 were not sustained, and measles vaccination coverage of preschool children remained around 60%.[32] In the mid- to late-1970s, changing measles epidemiology was evident with a significant proportion of cases occurring in school-aged children and outbreaks occurring in middle schools and high schools.[3,34,36]

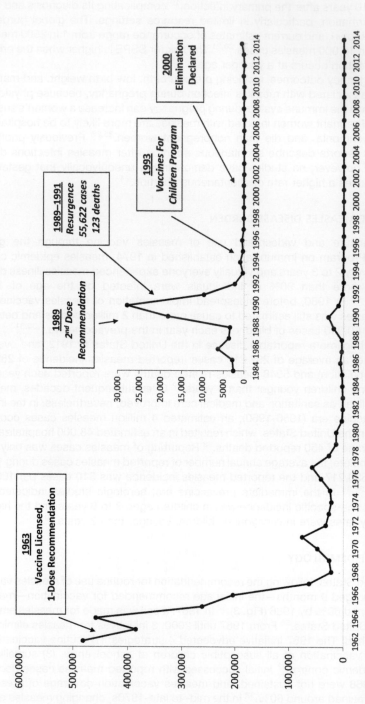

Fig. 3. Reported measles cases by year in United States, 1962-2014 (provisional total reported cases through December 31, 2014).

The second initiative focused efforts on increasing vaccination coverage at school entry and resulted in a decline of cases in the late 1970s and the 1980s. The great value of state-mandated and state-implemented vaccination requirements for school entry was demonstrated by studies that showed lower measles incidence in states with school entry requirements than in states without them and by a natural experiment that occurred during a measles outbreak in a divided city that spanned 2 states with different requirements.[3,37] Despite the focus on school requirements, coverage for preschool children aged 1 to 4 years remained less than 70% nationwide.[32,38]

During the 1980s, measles occurred mainly among unvaccinated preschool-aged children and school-aged students, most of who had received a single dose of measles vaccine.[36] Outbreaks in highly (>99%) vaccinated school populations suggested that a routine second dose of a measles-containing vaccine (specifically, measles-mumps-rubella [MMR] vaccine) was needed for all children, and this was recommended in 1989.[39] A measles resurgence during 1989-1991, with 53,685 reported cases resulting in an estimated 11,000 hospitalizations and 123 reported measles-related deaths, took the country by surprise.[40] In 1989, measles epidemiology was characterized by school-based outbreaks in predominantly vaccinated students, but as the resurgence progressed, the primary group affected was unvaccinated preschool-aged children living in poor urban areas in large cities.

The 1989-1991 measles resurgence highlighted the importance of delivering the first measles vaccine dose on time and tracking coverage in the preschool age group.[40] The resurgence also exposed the disparity in burden of disease and inequity of vaccination coverage among communities and led to sustained funding commitments to achieve measles elimination objectives, including improved access to vaccines through the Vaccines for Children's Program (the third initiative).[38] By the mid-1990s, first-dose measles vaccine coverage among children aged 19 to 35 months had reached 90% and states rapidly implemented second-dose school requirements. Accordingly, annual reported measles cases declined from 27,786 in 1990 to 508 in 1996 and remained less than 150 (incidence <1 per million) through the rest of the 1990s.[41] In 2000, a panel of experts in the United States was convened to review measles epidemiology, distribution of measles genotypes, population immunity, and adequacy of measles surveillance, and they concluded that measles was no longer endemic in the United States.[42]

The postelimination era in the United States has been characterized by importations of measles, with outbreaks of varying magnitudes occurring every year. During the first decade after elimination (2001-2010), a median of 60 cases a year were reported, and the largest outbreak had 34 cases.[43–45] However, during 2011-2014, the number of reported annual measles cases increased, with a median of 205 and range of 55 to 644 (**Fig. 4**) (Centers for Disease Control and Prevention [CDC], unpublished data, 2014). In 2014, an outbreak occurred with 382 reported measles cases, primarily among Amish communities in Ohio (CDC, unpublished data, 2014).[46] In the postelimination era, the vast majority of patients with measles are either unvaccinated or do not know their vaccination status and a high proportion of unvaccinated persons who are eligible for vaccination have chosen not to vaccinate themselves or their children because of their personal or religious beliefs.[4,47–49]

Globally, 279,776 measles cases were reported in 2013; however, measles is known to be grossly underreported and the disease burden was likely 8 million to 13 million cases (**Fig. 5**).[50,51] Disease modeling using surveillance and other data inputs are used to estimate annual global and regional measles mortality.[52] Following increasing vaccination coverage and measles elimination efforts, estimated measles cases and deaths have decreased substantially (**Fig. 6**). During 2000-2013, annual reported

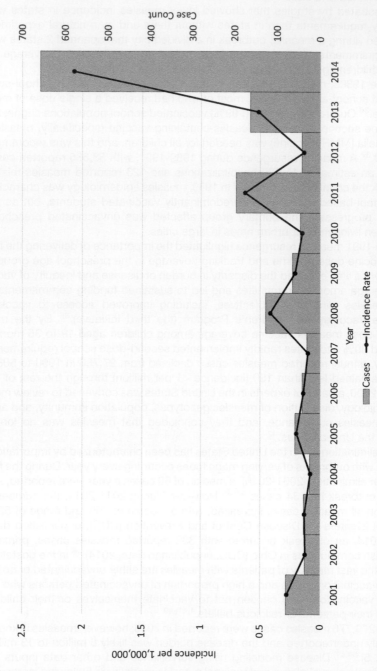

Fig. 4. Reported measles cases and incidence by year in the postelimination era in United States, 2001-2014 (provisional total reported cases through December 31, 2014).

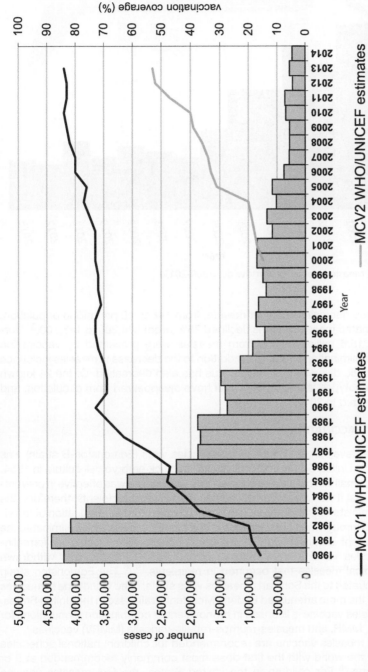

Fig. 5. Global number of reported measles cases (cases of measles reported to the WHO and the United Nations Children's Fund [UNICEF] through the Joint Reporting Form) and estimated coverage with the first and second dose of measles-containing vaccine (MCV; MCV1, first dose of MCV in routine immunization; MCV2, second dose of MCV in routine immunization. MCV2 estimates available from 2000 when global data collection started; however, some countries introduced the vaccine earlier. WHO/UNICEF MCV coverage estimates for 2014 not available as of July 9, 2015) through routine services, 1980-2014.

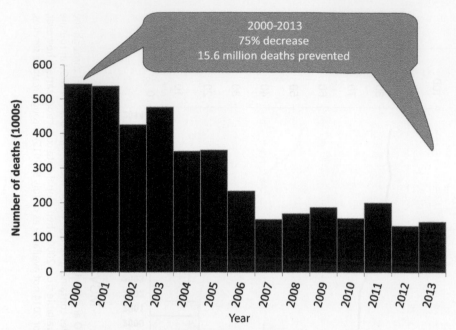

Fig. 6. Estimated measles mortality worldwide, 2000-2013.

measles incidence decreased 72% worldwide, from 146 to 40 per million population, and annual estimated measles deaths declined 75%, from 544,200 to 145,700.[53] During 2000-2013, 15.6 million deaths from measles were prevented by vaccination through measles elimination efforts.[53] In addition to the decrease in measles incidence globally, the genetic diversity of measles virus has also decreased. Of the 24 known measles virus genotypes, approximately half have disappeared from circulation, and only 8 were detected in 2014.[9]

PREVENTION BY VACCINATION

Measles vaccine development began when measles virus (Edmonston-B strain) was first isolated in the United States and propagated in chick embryo cell culture in 1954. In the late 1950s, small clinical studies showed that the vaccine was effective in preventing measles but that it was reactogenic, causing rash in most recipients; therefore, the vaccine was administered with immunoglobulin. However, further attenuation of the virus was achieved through multiple passages in chick embryo cells, which eliminated the need for concurrent administration of gamma globulin with vaccine. A formalin-inactivated measles vaccine was available during 1963-1968 but was withdrawn because of atypical measles that occurred in recipients.[15,16] The Edmonston strain was further attenuated to the Schwartz measles virus strain, used worldwide in measles vaccines, and to the more attenuated Enders (Moraten) strain used in the United States. Worldwide, measles vaccine is licensed in monovalent or combination formulations for measles-rubella, MMR, and measles-mumps-rubella-varicella (MMRV) vaccines.

Two doses of measles vaccine are recommended for children; national schedules vary throughout the world with the first dose most commonly recommended at 9 or 12 months of age.[28] For children in the United States, the first measles vaccine dose is recommended at 12 to 15 months of age and the second dose at 4 to 6 years of age or at least 28 days after the first dose (**Box 1**).[54] Vaccine recommendations may differ during outbreaks and before international travel.

Box 1
Prevention of measles: Recommendations from the ACIP, United States, 2013

Children and adolescents[a]

- Every office visit should be used as an opportunity to provide measles vaccine for unvaccinated eligible children. Delays in vaccination may result in infection from measles if exposed to the virus.
- Routine first dose at 12 to 15 months. The first dose should be administered as soon as possible upon reaching 12 months.
- Routine second dose at 4 to 6 years or at an earlier age provided the interval between the first and second dose is more than 28 days
- Catch-up vaccination as needed
- For children who travel abroad, a dose of MMR vaccine is recommended for infants aged 6 to 11 months and 2 appropriately spaced vaccine doses are recommended for children aged 12 months or older. Infants who receive a dose at the age from 6 to 11 months need to receive 2 valid MMR vaccine doses after their first birthday.
- All family and other close contacts of immunocompromised persons aged 12 months or older should receive 2 doses of MMR vaccine unless they have other evidence of measles immunity.

Adults

- Adults born in 1957 or later should receive at least 1 dose of MMR vaccine unless they have other acceptable evidence of immunity
- Health care personnel, students at post–high-school educational facilities, and international travelers should be protected with 2 appropriately spaced MMR vaccine doses unless they have other acceptable evidence of immunity.

During measles outbreaks

- If outbreaks affect preschool-aged children or adults with community-wide transmission, a second dose should be considered for children aged 1 to 4 years or adults who have received 1 dose.
- If outbreaks involve infants younger than 12 months with ongoing risk for exposure, infants aged 6 months or older can be vaccinated.
- Health care facilities should recommend 2 doses of MMR vaccine at the appropriate interval for unvaccinated health care personnel who lack laboratory evidence of measles, mumps, or rubella immunity or laboratory confirmation of disease, regardless of the birth year.

[a] Evidence of immunity from measles disease is rare in US-born children. Most children have evidence from age-appropriate vaccination. Vaccination is not needed if children have laboratory confirmation of disease or laboratory evidence of immunity. For details on evidence of immunity for adults and for health care personnel, consult Advisory Committee on Immunization Practices (ACIP) guidance. Vaccination recommendations during outbreaks differ from routine recommendations for health care personnel.[54]

Contraindications and Precautions

- Contraindications for MMR and MMRV vaccines include history of anaphylactic reactions to neomycin, history of severe allergic reaction to any component of the vaccine, pregnancy, and immunosuppression. Allergy to egg is not a contraindication to vaccination. Children with human immunodeficiency virus infection who do not have severe immunosuppression should receive MMR vaccine, but not MMRV vaccine.[54,55]

- Precautions for MMR and MMRV vaccines include recent ($\leq$11 months) receipt of an antibody-containing blood product, concurrent moderate or severe illness with or without fever, history of thrombocytopenia or thrombocytopenic purpura, and tuberculin skin testing.[54]

Safety and Efficacy/Effectiveness

- Measles vaccine has been proved to be safe and effective. Adverse events may occur in the second week following vaccination, including fever and transient rash. Rare adverse events include immune thrombocytopenic purpura (approximately 1 in 30,000–40,000 doses) and febrile seizures (approximately 1 in 3000–4000 doses) following the first dose of measles or MMR vaccine in young children.[28,56] Persons who developed thrombocytopenia with a previous dose might develop thrombocytopenia with a subsequent dose of MMR vaccine; therefore, serologic evidence of immunity can be sought to determine whether or not an additional dose of MMR or MMRV vaccine is needed.[54] Another dose of vaccine may be given if serologic immunity is not found on testing. Among children aged 12 to 23 months who received the first dose of MMRV vaccine, an approximate 2-fold increased risk exists for febrile seizures compared with children aged 12 to 23 months who received MMR and varicella vaccines separately.[54,55,57–60] These seizures occurred 5 to 12 days after vaccination. No increased risk for febrile seizures was observed after vaccination with MMRV vaccine in children aged 4 to 6 years, compared with MMR and varicella vaccines administered separately.[60,61]
- Measles vaccine effectiveness is 93% following 1 dose administered at the age of 12 months or greater and 97% for 2 doses.[54]
- Measles-vaccine-induced immunity provides protection that is likely lifelong.[62] Although antibody levels decline over time, they remain above protective levels for most vaccinated persons and there is no consistent evidence that protection from measles declines among adults.[63] However, continued monitoring of duration of immunity and protection is important.
- Available measles vaccines must be given using a hypodermic needle and syringe and pose significant logistical drawbacks, particularly in resource-limited settings. Active research is ongoing to develop alternative delivery methods, including a microneedle patch for intradermal vaccination.[64,65]

PATIENT HISTORY

In the postelimination era, measles cases occur in unimmunized persons, primarily among those who travel abroad or are exposed to measles virus from infected travelers or during outbreaks that occur following measles virus importation. Clinicians should maintain awareness of patient vaccination status, have a high index of suspicion for measles and other vaccine-preventable diseases in patients who are unvaccinated, and educate parents on procedures to be followed if they or their child develops symptoms consistent with measles. These procedures should include steps to avoid exposing other patients to measles virus by calling the office before the visit to alert clinicians to the symptoms before arrival and by bringing the child into the office at the beginning or the end of the day. If a child presents with an illness clinically compatible with measles, a detailed patient history should be obtained (**Box 2**).

DIFFERENTIAL DIAGNOSIS

Physicians who trained in the United States before 1970 or during the measles resurgence during 1989-1991 may be familiar with diagnosing and managing measles

---

Box 2
Patient history—suspected measles

- Has the patient recently traveled abroad?

- Has the patient has been in contact with others who traveled abroad or with a known measles case, or is there a measles outbreak in the local community?

- Has the patient attended a recent mass gathering or been in situations where he or she might have come into contact with international visitors?

- Is vaccination status appropriate for age?[a]

- When did symptoms start (dates of onset) and how did they progress?
  o Fever
  o Cough (usually dry)
  o Coryza (runny nose)
  o Conjunctivitis (runny eyes)
  o Sore throat
  o Photophobia
  o Characteristics, location, and progression of the rash
  o Other symptoms such as ear pain or discharge, diarrhea, or respiratory distress

[a] *Note:* measles occurs in unvaccinated children, but being vaccinated does not preclude the diagnosis of measles.

---

cases. However, since 2000, most physicians in the United States have never diagnosed or treated a case of measles. Consequently, measles cases presenting in medical settings in recent years have been initially misdiagnosed as a variety of other conditions, including acute viral illness, dengue, scarlet fever, drug reaction, or Kawasaki disease. When measles goes unrecognized, failure to implement appropriate isolation procedures can lead to nosocomial infections. Because measles importations occur in the United States each year, physicians should keep measles in their differential diagnosis of febrile rash illness, particularly if the patient history includes traveling recently, being unvaccinated, or residing in a community with a measles outbreak. Early diagnosis and confirmation is important to provide appropriate treatment and institute public health responses, including isolation of cases and quarantining of contacts who lack evidence of measles immunity, to interrupt continuing measles virus transmission.

DIAGNOSTIC AND LABORATORY TESTING

Measles virus can be cultured from clinical specimens; however, the most common methods used for confirmation of measles infection are detection of measles-specific IgM antibody using an enzyme-linked immunosorbent assay (ELISA) and detection of measles RNA by real-time reverse transcription polymerase chain reaction.[66] A serum sample and throat swab (or nasopharyngeal swab) should be obtained from suspected measles cases at the first contact. Urine samples may also contain virus, and collection of serum, throat swab, and urine specimens, when feasible to do so, can increase the likelihood of detecting virus. At the beginning of acute measles infection, ELISA can yield false-negative results, particularly within the first 3 days of rash onset when IgM antibody titers might not have risen to detectable levels. If a negative IgM result is obtained from serum collected within 72 hours of rash onset, a second serum sample should be collected at 72 hours or later after rash onset. As measles is a rare disease in the United States, even with very good laboratory tests available, false-positive results for measles IgM will occur. To minimize the problem of false-positive laboratory results, it is important to restrict case investigation and laboratory tests to patients most likely to have measles and, in addition, to collect specimens for detection of measles virus.

In vaccinated persons suspected of having measles, a negative IgM test result alone should not be used to rule out the diagnosis.[66] Tests for rise in IgG antibody levels between acute and convalescent specimens using quantitative or semi-quantatative methods or avidity testing may be helpful in certain situations. Virus detection or culture allows for measles virus genotyping and sequencing. Phylogenetic analyses and molecular epidemiology help efforts to monitor measles virus transmission pathways in populations and to verify elimination of endemic measles virus strains.[6]

THERAPEUTIC OPTIONS AND CASE MANAGEMENT

No specific antiviral therapies exist for measles; therefore, case management is focused on supportive care and prevention and treatment of complications and secondary infections. Measles cases should be treated for fever and other symptoms and for complications, including use of antibiotics for secondary bacterial infections. In the United States, children with severe measles, such as those who are hospitalized, should receive vitamin A; in other settings, treatment guidelines recommend vitamin A for all measles cases.[22,28] Measles virus is susceptible in vitro to ribavirin; however, no controlled trials have been conducted, and ribavirin is not approved by the US Food and Drug Administration for treatment of measles.

PROSPECTS OF ERADICATION AND ERADICATION STRATEGIES

The feasibility and benefits of achieving measles eradication have long been established.[67,68] In July 2010, an expert advisory panel convened by the WHO concluded that measles can and should be eradicated, and these conclusions have since been endorsed by the WHO Strategic Advisory Group of Experts and the World Health Assembly (WHA).[69] However, an eradication goal with a target date has yet to be adopted.

The Global Vaccine Action Plan (GVAP) is the key global document that provides the vision statement and serves as the guide for global immunization efforts in the world today. The GVAP was developed by global partners through the Decade of Vaccines project, largely funded by the Bill and Melinda Gates Foundation. In 2012, the WHA endorsed the GVAP with the objective to eliminate measles in 5 WHO regions by 2020; all 6 WHO regions have a goal for measles elimination by 2020 or earlier.[70] In 2012, the Measles & Rubella Initiative, a global partnership established in 2001 by 5 core partners, the American Red Cross, the US CDC, the United Nations Foundation, United Nations Children's Fund, and the WHO, launched the 2012-2020 Global Measles and Rubella Strategic Plan, with goals aligned to the GVAP.[30,53] Full implementation of the recommended strategies along with substantial investments in strengthening health systems and achieving equitable access to vaccination services will lead to the achievement of regional measles elimination goals and the eventual goal of global measles eradication.

CHALLENGES AND OPPORTUNITIES

Despite tremendous achievements in global measles control, measles virus still circulates, causing infections, severe disease, and death. Because measles virus is highly contagious, high levels of population measles immunity are needed to interrupt measles virus transmission. Measles vaccine is very effective, and high immunity levels can be achieved with very high (>95%) 2-dose vaccine coverage in children and by offering vaccine to susceptible persons who may have missed out on exposure to measles or vaccination. National and global commitment is critical to achieve measles elimination and eradication—a world without measles.

In the United States, measles elimination has been maintained for more than 15 years, but challenges remain. Despite national 1-dose coverage levels of 92%, one child in 12 is not vaccinated on time, and considerable variability exists in state coverage estimates. Population immunity could be increased considerably by addressing missed opportunities for vaccination.[71] Importations of measles continue to test population immunity. The most frequent sources of measles importations are unvaccinated US travelers returning from abroad, with subsequent transmission among clusters of intentionally unvaccinated persons. Unvaccinated people put themselves and others, including infants and persons with medical contraindications to vaccination, at risk for measles and its complications. Studies at the state or lower levels suggest increasing rates of vaccine exemption at school entry.[72] In California, nonmedical immunization exemption rates at kindergarten entry have increased an average of 9.2% (95% confidence interval, 8.8–9.6) per year from 0.6% in 1994 to 2.3% in 2009.[73] In 2015, following a measles outbreak with more than 100 cases, California abolished nonmedical exemptions.[74] Measles outbreak response is costly and disruptive to public health departments and hospitals.[75,76]

Globally, measles outbreaks continue in all regions of the world, slowing progress toward achieving measles elimination goals. During April 2014-March 2015, 15 (8%) countries had measles incidence of more than 50 cases per million population and measles remained endemic in several large countries, including China, the Democratic Republic of the Congo, Ethiopia, India, Indonesia, Nigeria, and Pakistan. Outbreak investigations and surveillance data analysis have shown clearly that most reported measles cases were in patients who had received fewer than the 2 recommended doses and that measles continues to occur because of suboptimal vaccination coverage. In 2013, 21 million infants globally missed the routine first dose of measles-containing vaccine.[53] Funding shortfalls have hampered global efforts to fully implement elimination strategies.[77–79] To accelerate progress, national immunization programs and global partnerships should be strengthened to ensure effective program management and strategy implementation. Experience in the region of the Americas, including in the United States, has shown that evidence-based policies and strategic use of vaccines can lead to elimination.[80] To prevent measles virus importations and outbreaks in the United States and elsewhere, and to resume progress toward measles elimination globally, long-term stable financial investments and commitments are needed.[80–83]

REFERENCES

1. Wolfson LJ, Strebel PM, Gacic-Dobo M, et al. Has the 2005 measles mortality reduction goal been achieved? A natural history modelling study. Lancet 2007; 369(9557):191–200.
2. Murray CJL, Lopez AD, Mathers CD. The global epidemiology of infectious diseases. Geneva (Switzerland): World Health Organization; 2004.
3. Orenstein WA, Halsey NA, Hayden GF, et al. From the Center for Disease control: current status of measles in the United States, 1973–1977. J Infect Dis 1978; 137(6):847–53.
4. Centers for Disease Control and Prevention (CDC). Measles - United States, January 1-August 24, 2013. MMWR Morb Mortal Wkly Rep 2013;62(36):741–3.

5. Diamond JM. Guns, germs, and steel: the fates of human societies. New York: Norton; 1999.

6. Strebel P, Papania M, Fiebelkorn AP, et al. Chapter 20: Measles Vaccine Vaccines, 6th edition. Elsevier/Saunders, 2013, p. 352–87.

7. Cliff A, Haggett P, Smallman-Raynor M. Measles: an historical geography of a major human viral disease from global expansion to local retreat, 1840–1990. Oxford and Cambridge, Mass; Blackwell; 1993.

8. Enders JF. Propagation in tissue cultures of cytopathogenic agents from patients with measles. Adv Exp Med Biol 1954;86(2):277–86.

9. World Health Organisation. Measles virus nomenclature update: 2012. Wkly Epidemiol Rec 2012;87(9):73–81.

10. Rota PA, Brown K, Mankertz A, et al. Global distribution of measles genotypes and measles molecular epidemiology. J Infect Dis 2011;204(Suppl 1): S514–23.

11. Yanagi Y, Takeda M, Ohno S. Measles virus: cellular receptors, tropism and pathogenesis. J Gen Virol 2006;87(10):2767–79.

12. Tahara M, Takeda M, Shirogane Y, et al. Measles virus infects both polarized epithelial and immune cells by using distinctive receptor-binding sites on its hemagglutinin. J Virol 2008;82(9):4630–7.

13. McChesney MB, Miller CJ, Rota PA, et al. Experimental measles. I. Pathogenesis in the normal and the immunized host. Virology 1997;233(1):74–84.

14. Perry R, Halsey N. The clinical significance of measles: a review. J Infect Dis 2004;189(Suppl 1):S4–16.

15. Fulginiti VA, Eller JJ, Downie AW, et al. Altered reactivity to measles virus. Atypical measles in children previously immunized with inactivated measles virus vaccines. JAMA 1967;202(12):1075–80.

16. Brodsky AL. Atypical measles. Severe illness in recipients of killed measles virus vaccine upon exposure to natural infection. JAMA 1972;222(11):1415–6.

17. Miller DL. Frequency of complications of measles, 1963. Report on a national inquiry by the public health laboratory service in collaboration with the society of medical officers of health. Br Med J 1964;2(5401):75–8.

18. Griffin DE, Tselis AC, Booss J. Measles virus and the nervous system. Handb Clin Neurol 2014;123:577–90.

19. Campbell H, Andrews N, Brown KE, et al. Review of the effect of measles vaccination on the epidemiology of SSPE. Int J Epidemiol 2007;36(6):1334–48.

20. Bellini WJ, Rota JS, Lowe LE, et al. Subacute sclerosing panencephalitis: more cases of this fatal disease are prevented by measles immunization than was previously recognized. J Infect Dis 2005;192(10):1686–93.

21. Schönberger K, Ludwig M-S, Wildner M, et al. Epidemiology of subacute sclerosing panencephalitis (SSPE) in Germany from 2003 to 2009: a risk estimation. PLoS One 2013;8(7):e68909.

22. Kimberlin DW, Brady MT, Jackson MA, et al. Red Book: 2015 Report of the Committee on Infectious Diseases. 30th edition. Elk Grove Village (IL): American Academy of Pediatrics; 2015.

23. Packer AD. The influence of maternal measles (morbilli) on the unborn child. Med J Aust 1950;1(25):835–8.

24. Gershon AA, Marin M, Seward JF. Measles and mumps. In: Remington and Klein's infectious diseases of the fetus and newborn infant. 8th edition. Philadelphia: Elsevier; 2015. p. 675–723.

25. Rasmussen SA, Jamieson DJ. What obstetric health care providers need to know about measles and pregnancy. Obstet Gynecol 2015;126(1):163–70.

26. Ogbuanu IU, Zeko S, Chu SY, et al. Maternal, fetal, and neonatal outcomes associated with measles during pregnancy: Namibia, 2009–2010. Clin Infect Dis 2014; 58(8):1086–92.

27. Edmunds WJ, Gay NJ, Kretzschmar M, et al. The pre-vaccination epidemiology of measles, mumps and rubella in Europe: implications for modelling studies. Epidemiol Infect Dec 2000;125(3):635–50.

28. World Health Organization. Measles vaccines: WHO position paper. Wkly Epidemiol Rec 2009;84(35):349–60.

29. Langmuir AD. Medical importance of measles. Am J Dis Child 1962;103: 224–6.

30. World Health Organization. Global Measles and Rubella Strategic Plan 2012–2020. 2012. Available at: http://www.who.int/immunization/newsroom/Measles_Rubella_StrategicPlan_2012_2020.pdf. Accessed July 7, 2015.

31. Semba RD, Semba RD, Bloem MW, et al. Measles blindness. Surv Ophthalmol 2004;49(2):243–55.

32. Hinman A, Orenstein W, Papania M. Evolution of measles elimination strategies in the United States. J Infect Dis 2004;189(Suppl 1):S17–22.

33. Orenstein WA, Papania MJ, Wharton ME. Measles elimination in the United States. J Infect Dis 2004;189(Suppl 1):S1–3.

34. Guris D, Harpaz R, Redd SB, et al. Measles surveillance in the United States: an overview. J Infect Dis 2004;189(Suppl 1):S177–84.

35. Sencer DJ, Dull HB, Langmuir AD. Epidemiologic basis for eradication of measles in 1967. Public Health Rep 1967;82(3):253–6.

36. Centers for Disease Control and Prevention (CDC). Measles outbreak among vaccinated high school students–Illinois. MMWR Morb Mortal Wkly Rep 1984; 33(24):349–51.

37. Landrigan PJ. Epidemic measles in a divided city. JAMA 1972;221(6):567–70.

38. The measles epidemic. The problems, barriers, and recommendations. The National Vaccine Advisory Committee. JAMA 1991;266(11):1547–52.

39. Centers for Disease Control and Prevention (CDC). Measles prevention. MMWR Morb Mortal Wkly Rep 1989;38(Suppl 9):1–18.

40. Atkinson WL, Orenstein WA, Krugman S. The resurgence of measles in the United States, 1989–1990. Annu Rev Med 1992;43:451–63.

41. Papania MJ, Seward JF, Redd SB, et al. Epidemiology of measles in the United States, 1997–2001. J Infect Dis 2004;189(Suppl 1):S61–8.

42. Papania MJ, Orenstein WA. Defining and assessing measles elimination goals. J Infect Dis 2004;189(Suppl 1):S23–6.

43. Parker AA, Staggs W, Dayan GH, et al. Implications of a 2005 measles outbreak in Indiana for sustained elimination of measles in the United States. N Engl J Med 2006;355(5):447–55.

44. Fiebelkorn AP, Redd SB, Gallagher K, et al. Measles in the United States during the postelimination era. J Infect Dis 2010;202(10):1520–8.

45. United States National Report M, 2012. Documentation and Verification of Measles, Rubella and Congenital Rubella Syndrome Elimination In the Region of the Americas. 2012. Available at: http://www.cdc.gov/measles/downloads/report-elimination-measles-rubella-crs.pdf. Accessed September 7, 2015.

46. Gastañaduy P, Redd S, Fiebelkorn A, et al. Measles - United States, January 1-May 23, 2014. MMWR Morb Mortal Wkly Rep 2014;63(22):496–9.

47. Sugerman DE, Barskey AE, Delea MG, et al. Measles outbreak in a highly vaccinated population, San Diego, 2008: role of the intentionally undervaccinated. Pediatrics 2010;125(4):747–55.

48. Papania MJ, Wallace GS, Icenogle JP, et al. Elimination of endemic measles, rubella, and congenital rubella syndrome from the Western hemisphere: the US experience. JAMA Pediatr 2014;168(2):148–55.
49. Centers for Disease Control and Prevention (CDC). Update: measles–United States, January-July 2008. MMWR Morb Mortal Wkly Rep 2008;57(33):893–6.
50. Papania M, Strebel P. Measles surveillance: the importance of finding the tip of the iceberg. Lancet 2005;365(9454):100–1.
51. Davis SF, Strebel PM, Atkinson WL, et al. Reporting efficiency during a measles outbreak in New York City, 1991. Am J Public Health 1993;83(7):1011–5.
52. Simons E, Ferrari M, Fricks J, et al. Assessment of the 2010 global measles mortality reduction goal: results from a model of surveillance data. Lancet 2012; 379(9832):2173–8.
53. Perry R, Gacic Dobo M, Dabbagh A, et al. Progress toward regional measles elimination–worldwide, 2000–2013. MMWR Morb Mortal Wkly Rep 2014;63(45): 1034–8.
54. McLean H, Fiebelkorn A, Temte J, et al. Prevention of measles, rubella, congenital rubella syndrome, and mumps, 2013: summary recommendations of the Advisory Committee on Immunization Practices (ACIP). MMWR Recomm Rep 2013; 62(RR-04):1–34.
55. Marin M, Broder KR, Temte JL, et al. Use of combination measles, mumps, rubella, and varicella vaccine: recommendations of the Advisory Committee on Immunization Practices (ACIP). MMWR Recomm Rep 2010;59(RR-3):1–12.
56. Macartney KK, Gidding HF, Trinh L, et al. Febrile seizures following measles and varicella vaccines in young children in Australia. Vaccine 2015;33(11):1412–7.
57. Klein NP, Fireman B, Yih WK, et al. Measles-mumps-rubella-varicella combination vaccine and the risk of febrile seizures. Pediatrics 2010;126(1):e1–8.
58. Jacobsen SJ, Ackerson BK, Sy LS, et al. Observational safety study of febrile convulsion following first dose MMRV vaccination in a managed care setting. Vaccine 2009;27(34):4656–61.
59. Schink T, Holstiege J, Kowalzik F, et al. Risk of febrile convulsions after MMRV vaccination in comparison to MMR or MMR+V vaccination. Vaccine 2014; 32(6):645–50.
60. Ma SJ, Xiong YQ, Jiang LN, et al. Risk of febrile seizure after measles–mumps–rubella–varicella vaccine: a systematic review and meta-analysis. Vaccine 2015; 33(31):3636–49.
61. Klein NP, Lewis E, Baxter R, et al. Measles-containing vaccines and febrile seizures in children age 4 to 6 years. Pediatrics 2012;129(5):809–14.
62. Dine M, Hutchins S, Thomas A, et al. Persistence of vaccine-induced antibody to measles 26–33 years after vaccination. J Infect Dis 2004;189(Suppl 1):S123–30.
63. LeBaron CW, Beeler J, Sullivan BJ, et al. Persistence of measles antibodies after 2 doses of measles vaccine in a postelimination environment. Arch Pediatr Adolesc Med 2007;161(3):294–301.
64. Goodson JL, Chu SY, Rota PA, et al. Research priorities for global measles and rubella control and eradication. Vaccine 2012;30(32):4709–16.
65. Edens C, Collins ML, Goodson JL, et al. A microneedle patch containing measles vaccine is immunogenic in non-human primates. Vaccine 2015. http://dx.doi.org/ 10.1016/j.vaccine.2015.02.074.
66. Kutty P, Rota J, Bellini W, et al. Manual for surveillance of vaccine preventable diseases. 6th edition. In: CDC (editor). Chapter 7 measles. 2013. Available at: http:// www.cdc.gov/vaccines/pubs/surv-manual/chpt07-measles.pdf. Accessed September 7, 2015.

67. Robbins FC. Prospects for worldwide control of measles: discussion I. Rev Infect Dis 1983;5(3):619–20.

68. Dowdle W, Cochi S. The principles and feasibility of disease eradication. Vaccine 2011;29(Suppl 4):D70–3.

69. Strebel PM, Cochi SL, Hoekstra E, et al. A world without measles. J Infect Dis 2011;204(Suppl 1):S1–3.

70. Nguku PM, Sharif SK, Mutonga D, et al. An investigation of a major outbreak of Rift Valley fever in Kenya: 2006–2007. Am J Trop Med Hyg 2010; 83(2 Suppl):5–13.

71. Smith PJ, Marcuse EK, Seward JF, et al. Children and adolescents unvaccinated against measles: geographic clustering, parents' beliefs, and missed opportunities. Public Health Reports 2015;130(5):485–504.

72. Omer SB, Salmon DA, Orenstein WA, et al. Vaccine refusal, mandatory immunization, and the risks of vaccine-preventable diseases. N Engl J Med 2009; 360(19):1981–8.

73. Richards J, Wagenaar B, Van Otterloo J, et al. Nonmedical exemptions to immunization requirements in California: a 16-year longitudinal analysis of trends and associated community factors. Vaccine 2013;31(29):3009–13.

74. USA Today. Available at: http://www.usatoday.com/story/news/2015/06/30/california-vaccine-bill/29485063/. Accessed September 7, 2015.

75. Chen SY, Anderson S, Kutty PK, et al. Health care–associated measles outbreak in the United States after an importation: challenges and economic impact. J Infect Dis 2011;203(11):1517–25.

76. Ortega-Sanchez IR, Vijayaraghavan M, Barskey AE, et al. The economic burden of sixteen measles outbreaks on United States public health departments in 2011. Vaccine 2014;32(11):1311–7.

77. Centers for Disease Control and Prevention (CDC). Global measles mortality, 2000-2008. MMWR Morb Mortal Wkly Rep 2009;58(47):1321–6.

78. Masresha BG, Fall A, Eshetu M, et al. Measles mortality reduction and pre-elimination in the African region, 2001–2009. J Infect Dis 2011;204(Suppl 1): S198–204.

79. Shibeshi ME, Masresha BG, Smit SB, et al. Measles resurgence in southern Africa: challenges to measles elimination. Vaccine 2014;32(16):1798–807.

80. Orenstein W, Seib K. Mounting a good offense against measles. N Engl J Med 2014;371(18):1661–3.

81. The Measles & Rubella Initiative. Available at: http://www.measlesrubellainitiative. org/. Accessed September 7, 2015.

82. World Health Organisation. Global progress towards regional measles elimination, worldwide, 2000–2013. Wkly Epidemiol Rec 2014;89(46):509–16.

83. Enhancing the work of the Department of Health and Human Services national vaccine program in global immunization: recommendations of the National Vaccine Advisory Committee: approved by the National Vaccine Advisory Committee on September 12, 2013. Public Health Rep 2014;129(Suppl 3):12–85.

Approach to Immunization for the Traveling Child

Angela L. Myers, MD, MPH[a], John C. Christenson, MD[b],*

KEYWORDS

- International • Travel • Vaccines • Children • Yellow fever • Typhoid

KEY POINTS

- Children traveling to limited-resource countries are at risk of acquiring a vaccine-preventable disease, such as hepatitis A, measles, typhoid fever, and yellow fever.
- Children visiting friends and relatives are at the highest risk of acquiring a travel-related infection, such as typhoid fever.
- Assessment of routine childhood and adolescent vaccines, including influenza vaccine, should take place at the pretravel visit.
- The need for yellow fever vaccine should be assessed and provided to children 9 months or older who are traveling to an endemic country, even if not required for entry into the country.
- Japanese encephalitis and rabies vaccines are recommended for children traveling to high-risk areas.

INTRODUCTION

More than 1.1 billion persons traveled internationally in 2014. Approximately 4% were pediatric-age travelers. All regions of the world noted an increase in travel. Many countries with limited resources are endemic to typhoid fever, yellow fever, hepatitis A, and malaria. Measles transmission has been observed in high numbers in many countries, including in Europe. Travelers to countries in Southeast Asia are at a particular high risk of acquiring Japanese encephalitis virus (JEV) infection and rabies. Although the risk of illness related to international travel in children is not known, it is thought to be similar to their parents. Young children may be at even higher risk owing to receipt of fewer vaccines due to age, greater risk for dehydration when ill, and less robust immune response in some instances. Although there are no commercially available vaccines in

---

[a] Department of Pediatrics, Division of Pediatric Infectious Diseases, Children's Mercy Hospital, University of Missouri-Kansas City School of Medicine, 2401 Gillham Road, Kansas City, MO 64108, USA; [b] Pediatric Travel Medicine, Ryan White Center for Pediatric Infectious Disease and Global Health, Indiana University School of Medicine, Riley Hospital for Children at IU Health, 705 Riley Hospital Drive, RI-3032, Indianapolis, IN 46202, USA
* Corresponding author.
E-mail address: jcchrist@iu.edu

Infect Dis Clin N Am 29 (2015) 745–757
http://dx.doi.org/10.1016/j.idc.2015.07.001
0891-5520/15/$ – see front matter © 2015 Elsevier Inc. All rights reserved.
id.theclinics.com

the United States to protect against traveler's diarrhea and malaria, vaccines against many travel-acquired infections are available. In the United States, children are routinely vaccinated against hepatitis A and measles. However, although not routinely administered in the United States, vaccines against yellow fever, typhoid, rabies, and JE are recommended when traveling to endemic regions. Thus, an assessment of routine immunizations, as well as necessary travel immunizations, is imperative weeks or even months before international travel if possible. Consideration of accelerating the routine immunization schedule for the individual patient before international travel is important, as it allows for earlier development of necessary immunity and serves to complete the series in patients who may be away for extended periods of time to countries in which access to these vaccines may be limited.

IMMUNIZATION PRACTICES

For each administered vaccine, a Vaccine Information Statement (VIS) must be provided. They can be obtained from the Centers for Disease Control and Prevention (CDC) Web site (www.cdc.gov/vaccines/pubs/vis). Administered vaccines must be recorded in the traveler's clinic visit form, including injection site, dose, log numbers, and expiration dates. It should also be documented that potential vaccine side effects were discussed and that a VIS was provided.

Vaccines against typhoid fever, JEV, and yellow fever require special purchasing and are not routinely available in the offices of primary care physicians. Clinicians are required to have prior authorization from the state health department to administer yellow fever vaccine; an official stamp is needed. For most vaccines, storage requirements are similar to those of other vaccines. Practitioners must be familiar with administration routes and potential side effects. The primary care practitioner could administer some recommended vaccines, such as tetanus-diphtheria boosters, meningococcal vaccines for an adolescent, and hepatitis A for a 1-year-old. These are frequently covered by the traveler's primary insurance and would not require out-of-pocket payment (other than a copayment).

The routine immunization schedule is initiated at birth with hepatitis B vaccine. The routine vaccine series, including diphtheria, tetanus toxoid, and acellular pertussis (DTaP); Haemophilus influenzae type b; pneumococcal conjugate vaccine-13 valent (PCV13); hepatitis B; inactivated polio vaccine (IPV); and rotavirus is typically started at 2 months of age. The minimum age for immunization is 6 weeks for most of these vaccines. Recommendations for the use of routine vaccines against measles, mumps, pertussis, hepatitis B, diphtheria, and tetanus are discussed in great detail elsewhere (www.cdc.gov/vaccines/schedules/index.html). **Table 1** contains the minimum age required for initiation of vaccination.

ROUTINE IMMUNIZATIONS OF IMPORTANCE FOR TRAVELERS
Measles

Measles, mumps, and rubella vaccine (MMR) is an important part of the childhood immunization schedule, which is typically provided at 12 to 15 months and then a second dose at 4 to 5 years of age. However, the vaccine should be given to children 6 through 11 months of age who are traveling internationally. This vaccine dose does not count in the 2-dose series, and thus 2 vaccines after the age of 12 months and at least 28 days apart must be given after return to the United States. For children who are older than 12 months and have received their first dose of MMR, a second dose should be given before international travel, provided it has been 28 days since the previous dose. This dose can be counted for school entry.

Table 1
Minimum age for initiation of vaccination

Vaccine	Age
Hepatitis B	Birth
DTaP, IPV, Hib	6 wk
Pneumococcal conjugate	6 wk
Influenza, inactivated	6 mo
Influenza, live-attenuated	2 y
Measles-mumps-rubella	6 mo
Varicella	12 mo
Hepatitis A	12 mo or younger
Typhoid Vi injectable	2 y
Typhoid oral	6 y
Yellow fever	9 mo
Meningococcal conjugate	6 wk

Abbreviations: DTaP, acellular pertussis, Hib, *Haemophilus influenzae* type b; IPV, inactivated polio vaccine.

Data from Centers for Disease Control and Prevention. Epidemiology and Prevention of Vaccine-Preventable Diseases. Hamborsky J, Kroger A, Wolfe S, editors. 13th edition. Washington D.C. Public Health Foundation, 2015.

Most measles outbreaks in the United States have an international connection, and occur when an unimmunized visiting traveler brings measles into the United States, or when a US citizen travels to an endemic country (or a country experiencing an outbreak) and does not have protective immunity (eg, unvaccinated, vaccine nonresponder, or immune compromised). Imported measles is able to spread easily in communities in which there is a high rate of unvaccinated individuals. Measles remains common in many parts of the world, including Europe, Asia, the Pacific islands, and Africa. Thus, travelers to these regions need to ensure they are adequately immunized before travel.[1,2]

Polio

The CDC and the World Health Organization (WHO) have been involved in attempting to eliminate polio worldwide since 1988. The incidence of polio has dropped more than 99% since that time, but areas of risk still exist. Polio transmission has never been interrupted in 2 countries: Afghanistan and Pakistan. An additional 8 previously polio-free countries reported spread of wild poliovirus in 2014: Cameroon, Ethiopia, Equatorial Guinea, Iraq, Israel, Nigeria, Somalia, and Syria. Although there have not been any polio cases that originated within the United States since 1979, travelers have brought the virus (wild and vaccine-derived strains) into the country. Thus, it is important to ensure adequate immunization before travel. For infants and children who are traveling to a country in which there was polio transmission in the past 12 months, the immunization series should be completed before departure. This may be done in an accelerated fashion, with the first dose given at 6 weeks, followed by the second and third doses each 4 weeks apart, and the fourth dose 6 months after the third dose. If the accelerated schedule cannot be completed before departure, it should be completed in the destination country. The polio vaccination status of adult travelers also should be assessed. For adults who are known to be current with their polio series, a 1-time dose of IPV should be given before travel. Adults who are known to be unvaccinated, undervaccinated, or their vaccine status is unknown should receive a full vaccine series before departure. This series includes 2 doses separated by 4 weeks and a third dose at least 6 months after the second dose. In May 2014, the International Health Regulations Emergency Committee passed a resolution that countries known to be exporters of wild polioviruses, such Pakistan, implement a requirement that all residents and long-term visitors staying more than 4 weeks must receive an oral polio vaccine or IPV 4 weeks to 12 months before international travel (even if they have completed their primary series and are up-to-date according to their age). Documentation of this vaccine must appear on an International Certificate of Vaccination (yellow card).[3]

Pertussis

Pertussis is an important vaccine in the primary immunization series for children, and remains important throughout adolescence and into adulthood. The tetanus toxoid, reduced diphtheria toxoid, and acellular pertussis (Tdap) vaccine is part of the recommended adolescent immunization series and should be given between 11 and 12 years of age and before international travel. Older adolescents and adults who have not previously received Tdap vaccine should receive 1 dose before travel, even if they have received a tetanus toxoid (Td) vaccine recently. In recent years, there have been many case reports of international adoptees infecting contacts residing in their new communities.

Influenza

Infants and children are at an increased risk of influenza during international travel, especially when travel occurs during the peak influenza season and when travel occurs to Asia. Exposures occur at the home of relatives and friends, and during flight. All children 6 months of age or older should be vaccinated against influenza. For travel to countries in the Southern Hemisphere, a different vaccine may be required, and should be sought out in the destination country, because the antigen composition may differ with that used in the Northern Hemisphere.

HEALTH PREPARATION FOR LONG-STAY TRAVELERS

The risk of illness or injury increases as the duration of travel increases. Special consideration should be given for families who are planning long stays ($\geq$6 months) in limited-resource countries. Among the issues that should be discussed during the pretravel consultation should include how to access care at their destination, especially vaccines. It is especially important for families to understand that establishment of a primary care physician for their child is essential during long-term stays.

Several resources (**Box 1**) are available to help families establish medical care before traveling, including the US Department of State, the International Society of Travel Medicine, American Society of Tropical Medicine and Hygiene, and the International Association for Medical Assistance to Travelers. Specific embassies and

---

Box 1
Internet sites listing medical care providers by country

www.usembassy.gov

www.istm.org

www.iamat.org/doctors_clinics.cfm

www.astmh.org

consulates within the country of travel, hotel physicians, and credit card companies also may be able to provide guidance. Some supplemental medical insurance plans provide a 24-hour hotline to locate local care providers for travelers who purchased plans before travel.

RECOMMENDED TRAVEL IMMUNIZATIONS
Hepatitis A

Hepatitis A vaccine (HAV) is routinely administered to children who are 12 months of age or older. Since the introduction of HAVs, the incidence of hepatitis A among travelers has decreased significantly (**Table 2**). HAV is one of the most frequently administered vaccines. HAVs are highly protective and are well tolerated. Travel remains a key risk factor for the spread of hepatitis A.[4,5] Hepatitis A vaccination is recommended for all travel to countries with limited resources. HAVs appear to be immunogenic at all ages. After the administration of the 2 doses that comprised the series, protection is estimated to last at least 30 years. The accelerated schedule of the combined hepatitis A-B vaccine is useful in previously unvaccinated adults planning international travel and/or international adoption (see **Table 2**). This schedule requires 4 doses, and immunogenicity after 3 doses is $\geq$99.9%.

Before the licensing of HAVs, protection for travelers was achieved through the intramuscular administration of human serum immune globulin (IG). Unfortunately, protection was short-lived and only partially protective in some individuals. Travelers expecting prolonged stays in high-risk regions, required readministration every 3 to

Table 2
Hepatitis A vaccines for infants, children, adolescents, and adults

Vaccine/Type of Patient	Dose (mL)	No. of Doses	Schedule
Hepatitis A vaccines			
1–18 y of age			
Havrix (GSK Biologicals, Middlesex, UK), 720 ELU	0.5	2	0, 6–12 mo later
Vaqta (Merck & Co, Kennilworth, NJ, USA), 25 U	0.5	2	0, 6–18 mo later
>19 y of age			
Havrix (GSK Biologicals, Middlesex, UK), 1440 ELU	1.0	2	0, 6–12 mo later
Vaqta (Merck & Co, Kennilworth, NJ, USA), 50 U	1.0	2	0, 6–18 mo later
Hepatitis A and B vaccine			
Adults >18 y of age			
Twinrix (GSK Biologicals, Middlesex, UK)[a]	1.0	3–4[b-g]	0, 1 and 6 mo or 0, 7, 21–30 d + 12 mo later

Abbreviations: ELU, enzyme-linked immunosorbent assay units; U, Antigen units (each unit equivalent to 1 µg of viral protein).
  [a] Combination vaccine: hepatitis B (Engerix B, 20 µg) + hepatitis A (Havrix, 720 ELU).
  [b] Recombivax HB, 5 µg or Engerix B, 10 µg.
  [c] First dose is given in combination with hepatitis B-immune globulin.
  [d] Recombivax HB, 10 µg or Engerix B, 20 µg.
  [e] Special formulation of Recombivax HB.
  [f] Adult formulation of Recombivax HB.
  [g] Two 1.0 mL doses of Engerix B.

5 months (**Table 3**). The CDC recommends that all travelers younger than 12 months receive a single dose of IG (0.02–0.06 mL/kg).[6] However, some experts question this practice. IG is expensive, of short protection, and is difficult to find. In addition, hepatitis A in children younger than 3 years is an anicteric infection and frequently asymptomatic. When ill, it tends to be mild, with nonspecific complaints and findings. Thus, some question the need for immunization of young infants.

A major reason for considering vaccinating a young infant is to protect older susceptible individuals who may come in contact with a contagious asymptomatic infant during or after travel. These infants may infect an accompanying adult or relative after returning to a developed country. The scenario is plausible, because frequently parents bring their young children in for vaccination, but elect not to receive vaccines themselves. International adoptees are known to infect susceptible contacts.[7–9] To maximize protection, vaccination of infants born from seronegative mothers could be the focus, but hepatitis A antibody titers would have to be measured. Maternal antibodies against hepatitis A virus may blunt the infant's immune response. Although titers may still be in the protective range, they are lower than those observed in infants born from seronegative mothers.[10] If the mother's titer is negative, then you could vaccinate the infant. However, in some settings, serologic testing followed by vaccination is not cost-effective. Vaccinating all infants could be more economical. Although the use of HAV in young infants has been found to be safe, its administration has not been approved by the Food and Drug Administration (FDA) and is not endorsed by the Advisory Committee on Immunization Practices.

Immunocompromised persons can receive hepatitis A vaccination, especially if considering travel to countries with limited resources. Although approximately 75% will develop antibodies, the robustness of this response is influenced by the degree and type of immunosuppression.[11] Because of the variability of immune responses, an antibody titer after completion of the vaccine series appears reasonable.

Typhoid Fever

Enteric fever is prevalent worldwide, but it is only in those countries in which improvements in public health and sanitation have been implemented where the incidence of typhoid and paratyphoid fever is low. Enteric fever is a common systemic infection observed in limited-resource countries. It is caused by *Salmonella enterica*, which includes 2 serotypes, *Salmonella typhi* and *Salmonella paratyphi* A, B, or C. Adherence to the exclusive consumption of clean water and low-risk foods decreases the frequency of typhoid fever infections. Infections may lead to complications, such as intestinal hemorrhage, perforation, and prolonged fevers. Although mortality in travelers is low, morbidity is high. Travel to South Asia (India, Pakistan, Nepal, Sri Lanka, and

Table 3			
Use of immunoglobulin preparations to prevent hepatitis A			
Clinical Scenario	**Dose[a]**	**No. of Doses**	**Comments**
Preexposure, <12 mo of age[b]	0.02 mL/Kg	1	IG is administered deep into large muscle mass. Protects up to 3 mo.
	0.06 mL/kg	1	For travel ≥3 mo duration. Repeat every 5 mo if exposures to hepatitis A continues.
Postexposure[b]	0.02 mL/kg	1	To be given within 2 wk of exposure.

[a] Immune globulin (IG). Not more than 5 mL at one site (adults), 3 mL in infants and small children.
[b] For children ≥1 year of age: if unvaccinated, use hepatitis A vaccine (see **Table 2**).

Bangladesh) poses the highest risk of infection. Parts of Africa and Latin America also are affected, but at a lower frequency. Travel to limited-resource countries throughout the world comes with a recommendation for vaccination. Visiting friends and relatives, and prolonged stays, especially in rural regions, pose a greater risk of infection. Various typhoid fever vaccines are commercially available around the world. An injectable formulation, such as Vi capsular polysaccharide vaccine and an oral form of the live, attenuated vaccine (Ty21a), are available in the United States (**Table 4**).[12] Vaccine efficacy is variable, ranging from 19% to 96%, with an average vaccination efficacy closer to 50%. In a recent study from the United Kingdom, overall effectiveness was 65%.[13] There is no effective licensed vaccine against S paratyphi; however, the oral typhoid vaccine Ty21a demonstrates some cross-protection against S paratyphi.[14]

Yellow Fever

This viral infection is endemic to regions within sub-Saharan Africa and South America. It is estimated that the risk of acquiring yellow fever (YF) in unvaccinated travelers to West Africa is approximately 10 to 50 cases per 100,000 visits over a 2-week exposure. Estimates of disease after travel to the Amazon Basin of South America are lower. YF will be asymptomatic or mild in approximately 50% to 85% of infections, but the case fatality rate varies between 5% and 50%, and cases among unvaccinated travelers are well-recognized. The YF vaccine is highly effective and generally safe. However, the first dose may rarely be associated with potentially fatal viscerotropic and neurologic disease. These severe adverse events are mostly observed in persons 60 years and older. Because YF vaccine is a live-attenuated vaccine, its use is contraindicated in immunocompromised individuals. The vaccine is also contraindicated in infants younger than 4 months. Lower risk for complications is observed in infants 9 months of age or older. Clinicians are cautioned to only vaccinate infants between the ages of 6 and 8 months if travel cannot be postponed to a later date. Under these circumstances, the benefits of the vaccine must outweigh the potential risk of the vaccine. However, limited published data show that the vaccine is immunogenic and well tolerated in this group.[15]

Table 4 Typhoid vaccines	
Oral typhoid vaccine Ty21a	For persons ≥6 y of age. Series: 4 doses; 1 capsule every other day (days 0, 2, 4, and 6). Take with cool water, 1 h before meal. Must complete series at least 1 wk before exposure. Capsules must be refrigerated. Capsules should not be broken and contents mixed with food/water. This inactivates the vaccine. Should not be taken with antibiotics. Repeat 4-dose series every 5 y if exposure continues. Contraindicated in immunocompromised conditions. Potential side effects: nausea, abdominal pain, cramps, vomiting, fever, headaches, and rash.
Injectable polysaccharide typhoid vaccine	For persons ≥2 y of age. Single injection, 0.5 mL, intramuscular, deltoid. Single injection at least 2 wk before exposure. Thimerosal-free. Booster: every 2 y if exposure continues. Potential side effects: injection site pain, erythema and induration; occasional fever, flulike symptoms.

An analysis by a working group within WHO has shown the presence of neutralizing antibodies against YF in approximately 90% of YF vaccine recipients 16 to 19 years after vaccination, and often longer. Rather than having revaccination every 10 years, WHO is recommending once in a lifetime vaccination against YF.[16]

Meningococcal Disease

Epidemic meningococcal sepsis and meningitis is a serious problem in the sub-Saharan region of Africa. Specific serogroups, such as A and W135, have been responsible for epidemics in Burkina Faso, Mali, and Saudi Arabia. Preschool children accompanying their parents on the Hajj or traveling to sub-Saharan Africa should receive meningococcal vaccination before travel. In recent months, an epidemic of group C has been reported in Chad.

There are 6 FDA-approved vaccines in the market: 3 conjugated (2 quadrivalent, 1 bivalent vaccine combined with *H influenzae* type b antigen), a quadrivalent polysaccharide vaccine, and 2 group B vaccines (**Table 5**). A serogroup A meningococcal vaccine (MenAfrVac; Serum Institute of India, Ltd, Pune) has been used in Burkina Faso, Niger, and Mali with significant effectiveness. Quadrivalent conjugate meningococcal vaccines are administered routinely in the United States to children at 11 to 12 years of

Table 5
Meningococcal conjugate vaccines

Vaccine	Age Groups	Dosage	Route	Schedule
Meningococcal oligosaccharide diphtheria CRM$_{197}$ conjugate vaccine, MenACWY-CRM (Menveo, Novartis [Basel, Switzerland])[a,b]	2–12 mo	0.5 mL	IM	0, 2, 4, 10–13 mo
	7–23 mo	0.5 mL	IM	0, 3 mo (second dose administered in second year of life)
	2–55 y	0.5 mL	IM	1 dose
Meningococcal polysaccharide diphtheria toxoid conjugate vaccine, MenACWY-D (Menactra, Sanofi Pasteur, Lyon, France)[a,b]	9–23 mo	0.5 mL	IM	0, 3 mo
	2–55 y	0.5 mL	IM	1 dose
HibMenCY-TT (MenHibRix, GSK) *Haemophilus influenzae* type b-*Neisseria meningitidis* CY combination vaccine[c]	6 wk–18 mo	0.5 mL	IM	0, 2, 4, 10–13 mo
Group B meningococcal (Bexsero, Novartis [Basel, Switzerland] and Trumenba, Pfizer-Wyeth, NY, USA)	10–25 y	0.5 mL	IM	0, 30 d (Bexsero) 0, 2, and 6 mo (Trumenba)

Abbreviation: IM, intramuscular.
[a] If an infant is receiving vaccine before travel, 2 doses can be administered 8 weeks apart.
[b] Revaccination: Is recommended after 3 years for children previously vaccinated between the ages of 9 months and 6 years, and after 5 years for previously vaccinated persons 7–55 years of age. Revaccination is thereafter recommended every 5 years if continued risk exists.
[c] This vaccine is not generally recommended for travel to sub-Saharan Africa, a region where group A and W strains predominate.

age, with a recommended booster 5 years later. High-risk children can be vaccinated as young as 2 months of age. The meningococcal quadrivalent polysaccharide conjugate diphtheria toxoid vaccine (Menactra; Sanofi Pasteur, Lyon, France) has been licensed for use in high-risk infants as young as 9 months of age. A combination bivalent conjugate vaccine protective against serogroup C and Y and *H influenzae* type b has been licensed for use in high-risk infants as young as 2 months of age. The meningococcal conjugate CRM$_{197}$ vaccine is the only quadrivalent vaccine approved for use starting at 2 months of age because it does not interfere with antibody production by the pneumococcal conjugate vaccine. Due to the high risk of disease acquisition in young infants, consideration should be given to refrain from traveling to endemic areas with infants younger than 2 months of age.

Rabies

Rabies is a disease with high mortality and high exposure rate. Most reported cases of rabies occur in Africa and Asia. Most cases result from the bite of a rabid dog. In some countries, monkey bites are frequent. The administration of vaccines is prioritized based on the likelihood of exposure, incidence among travelers, severity of disease if infected, and available treatment. In the case of rabies, the availability of postexposure human rabies immune globulin (HRIG) and vaccine greatly influence the decision to vaccinate before travel. Cost consideration clearly influences the likelihood of vaccination. Although the incidence of rabies in a traveler is more than 1 per 1 million persons, the incidence of high-risk animal bites is significantly higher, approximately 1 per 100 travelers per month. A bite in an unvaccinated child in high-endemic regions of Southeast and South Asia would necessitate postexposure prophylaxis, and likely disruption in travel plans, if HRIG and vaccines are not locally available. Strong consideration should be given to vaccinate children, especially toddlers, visiting remote locations in high-risk areas of the globe with limited access to health care facilities. Unfortunately, only a small number of travelers receive preexposure prophylaxis before travel. In a study from New Zealand, children 5 to 15 years were at the highest risk of being bitten.[17] In a recent study from Australia, only 58.5% of bitten individuals received HRIG.[18] Only 9% received it abroad. The mean delay from injury to HRIG was 15 days, which is too late to provide protection during the 2-week window period from vaccination to development of protective antibody. Only 4% of international travelers received preexposure vaccination.

Global availability of rabies IG and vaccine can be quite variable from one region to another. In a global assessment performed by Jentes and colleagues,[19] in some regions of the world rabies IG and vaccines was seldom available, with tropical South America having the least access to HRIG and vaccines. When available, some countries had access to equine-derived IG, a product with a greater potential for adverse reactions, such as allergic reactions. **Table 6** has recommendations for preexposure and postexposure prophylaxis.

Japanese Encephalitis

Culex mosquitoes transmit the flavivirus JEV. Asymptomatic infection is common, with 1:200 developing clinical disease. Fewer than 1% of human JEV infections result in encephalitis. In endemic regions of Asia, JE is primarily a disease of children. Most adults have natural immunity after childhood infection. In most temperate areas of Asia, transmission mainly occurs during the warm season (May–October). In the tropics and subtropics of Asia, transmission occurs year-round. The rate of transmission intensifies during the rainy season.[20] Case fatality rate is 20% to 30%, and 30% to 50% of survivors suffer neurologic or psychiatric sequelae. Although there is no licensed antiviral therapy, the disease is vaccine-preventable.[21]

Table 6
Rabies immunizations

Vaccine/Product	Dose	Schedule	Route	Number of Doses
Preexposure immunization				
Human diploid cell vaccine (HDCV), Imovax (Sanofi Pasteur, Lyon, France)	1.0 mL	0, 7, and 21, or 28 d	IM	3
Purified chick embryo cell vaccine (PCEC), RabAvert (Novartis, Basel, Switzerland)	1.0 mL	0, 7, and 21, or 28 d	IM	3
Postexposure immunization: Not previously vaccinated				
Human rabies immune globulin (HRIG)	20 IU/kg body weight	Once	Infiltrated at bite (if possible). Remainder IM	1
HDCV or PCEC	1.0 mL	0, 3, 7, 14 d (28 if immunocompromised)[a]	IM	4–5
Postexposure immunization: Previously vaccinated[b]				
HDCV or PCEC	1.0 mL	0, 3 d	IM	2

Abbreviation: IM, intramuscular.
[a] An antibody titer is recommended 1 month after receiving the fifth dose.
[b] If previously vaccinated, HRIG is not required.

Risk for most travelers is very low. The overall estimated incidence for persons from nonendemic countries traveling to Asia is fewer than 1 case per 1 million travelers. However, the risk varies depending on the travel destination, duration of travel, season, and planned activities. Extensive outdoor or nighttime exposure in rural areas during periods of active transmission poses the greatest risk of infection. Travel restricted to major urban areas is of minimal risk for JE. Risk is much higher for expatriates and travelers who stay for prolonged periods in rural areas with active JEV transmission, where the incidence of disease is 5 to 50 cases per 100,000 children per year. Stays longer than 1 month pose the highest risk, but one-third of cases occurred in endemic areas with travel of less than 1 month's duration. Approximately 60% of these cases occurred in tourists.

JEV vaccine (Ixiaro; Intercell, Vienna, Austria) in young children is highly immunogenic (95.7%).[22] The vaccine is well tolerated. **Table 7** contains information of dosage and schedule for children and adults.

TRAVEL VACCINES NOT AVAILABLE IN THE UNITED STATES
Bacille Calmette-Guérin

The Bacille Calmette-Guérin (BCG) vaccine is widely used in many countries around the world with high rates of endemic tuberculosis (TB). It is used to prevent childhood tuberculous meningitis and miliary disease. Because BCG vaccine is not

Table 7				
Japanese encephalitis vaccine, inactivated, Ixiaro				
Age Group	Dosage	Route	Schedule	Comments
≥2 mo to <3 y	3 µg (0.25 mL)	IM	0, 28 d	A booster is recommended for adults ≥1 y
≥3 y	6 µg (0.5 mL)			after primary series. There is no specific
Adults	6 µg (0.5 mL)			data in children.

Abbreviation: IM, intramuscular.

recommended for routine use in the United States, its availability is almost nonexistent. Parents taking their young infants to high-endemic countries may want to vaccinate their children at the destination country.

Tick-Borne Encephalitis

Tick-borne encephalitis vaccine provides protection from the most common arthropod-transmitted viral infection in Europe and eastern Asia. This disease closely resembles YF, West Nile virus, and dengue virus in the Flaviviridae family and is caused by the bite of the *Ixodes* tick and sometimes by ingestion of unpasteurized dairy products. European countries with the highest incidence include Germany, Switzerland, Austria, the Czech Republic, Slovakia, Hungary, Slovenia, the Baltic countries, Poland, parts of Scandinavia, European Russia, and Northern Japan. Transmission occurs from April through November, with a bimodal peak in early and late summer. Most cases occur at elevations less than 2500 feet and the overall risk of disease is estimated at 1:10,000 person-months of exposure. Most cases occur in forested areas, and the risk is negligible for those who are staying in urban areas and who do not consume unpasteurized dairy products. There are multiple age-specific vaccines licensed in Europe and Canada. Although the tick-borne encephalitis vaccine is not available in the United States and is not routinely recommended for people traveling to endemic areas, it can be considered by individuals who are planning long stays and will have high-risk exposures (eg, adventure travel or camping in forested areas).[23]

Pediatric Hepatitis A/B Vaccine

The combined hepatitis A/B vaccine for children, known as Twinrix Junior (GlaxoSmithKline), is available in Canada for children aged 1 to 18 years as a 3-dose series given at 0, 1, and 6 months. This vaccine is similar to the Twinrix vaccine available in the United States for adults, at half the adult dose. The vaccine has shown good efficacy in children at 100% seroprotection for hepatitis A and greater than 96% for hepatitis B. A rapid schedule is available in the United States for adults who have imminent travel and are not currently protected. The vaccine is given on days 0, 7, 21, and then again at 1 year.

FUTURE TRAVEL VACCINES

In recent years, new developments in vaccine technology have introduced into clinical trials vaccines against dengue fever and malaria.[24–26] Early results are promising. A conjugate Vi polysaccharide typhoid vaccine was found to be effective in preventing severe disease in an endemic area.[27]

REFERENCES

1. Hagmann SH, Christenson JC. Measles and the risk posed by international travelers at the time of elimination or post-elimination. Travel Med Infect Dis 2015;13:1–2.

2. Jost M, Luzi D, Metzler S, et al. Measles associated with international travel in the region of the Americas, Australia and Europe, 2001-2013: a systematic review. Travel Med Infect Dis 2015;13:10–8.
3. Wallace GS, Seward JF, Pallansch MA, et al. Interim CDC guidance for polio vaccination for travel to and from countries affected by wild poliovirus. MMWR Morb Mortal Wkly Rep 2014;63:591–4.
4. Kumbang J, Ejide S, Tedder RS, et al. Outbreak of hepatitis A in an extended family after importation by non-immune travellers. Epidemiol Infect 2012;140:1813–20.
5. Faillon S, Martinot A, Hau I, et al. Impact of travel on the seroprevalence of hepatitis A in children. J Clin Virol 2013;56:46–51.
6. Brunett GW. Centers for Disease Control and Prevention. CDC health information for international travel 2016. New York: Oxford University Press; 2016.
7. Fischer GE, Teshale EH, Miller C, et al. Hepatitis A among international adoptees and their contacts. Clin Infect Dis 2008;47:812–4.
8. Pelletier AR, Mehta PJ, Burgess DR, et al. An outbreak of hepatitis A among primary and secondary contacts of an international adoptee. Public Health Rep 2010;125:642–6.
9. Sweet K, Sutherland W, Ehresmann K, et al. Hepatitis A infection in recent international adoptees and their contacts in Minnesota, 2007-2009. Pediatrics 2011; 128:e333–8.
10. Bell BP, Negus S, Fiore AE, et al. Immunogenicity of an inactivated hepatitis A vaccine in infants and young children. Pediatr Infect Dis J 2007;26:116–22.
11. Garcia Garrido HM, Wieten RW, Grobusch MP, et al. Response to hepatitis A vaccination in immunocompromised travelers. J Infect Dis 2015;212(3):378–85.
12. Jackson BR, Iqbal S, Mahon BMP, et al. Updated recommendations for the use of typhoid vaccine–Advisory Committee on Immunization Practices, United States, 2015. MMWR Morb Mortal Wkly Rep 2015;64:305–8.
13. Wagner KS, Freedman JL, Andrews NJ, et al. Effectiveness of the typhoid Vi vaccine in overseas travelers from England. J Travel Med 2015;22:87–93.
14. Pakkanen SH, Kantele JM, Kantele A. Cross-reactive gut-directed immune response against Salmonella enterica serovar Paratyphi A and B in typhoid fever and after oral Ty21a typhoid vaccination. Vaccine 2012;30:6047–53.
15. Osei-Kwasi M, Dunyo SK, Koram KA, et al. Antibody response to 17D yellow fever vaccine in Ghanaian infants. Bull World Health Organ 2001;79:1056–9.
16. Gotuzzo E, Yactayo S, Cordova E. Efficacy and duration of immunity after yellow fever vaccination: systematic review on the need for a booster every 10 years. Am J Trop Med Hyg 2013;89:434–44.
17. Shaw MT, O'Brien B, Leggat PA. Rabies postexposure management of travelers presenting to travel health clinics in Auckland and Hamilton, New Zealand. J Travel Med 2009;16:13–7.
18. Kardamanidis K, Cashman P, Durrheim DN. Travel and non-travel associated rabies post exposure treatment in New South Wales residents, Australia, 2007-2011: a cross-sectional analysis. Travel Med Infect Dis 2013;11:421–6.
19. Jentes ES, Blanton JD, Johnson KJ, et al. The global availability of rabies immune globulin and rabies vaccine in clinics providing direct care to travelers. J Travel Med 2013;20:148–58.
20. Shlim DR, Solomon T. Japanese encephalitis vaccine for travelers: exploring the limits of risk. Clin Infect Dis 2002;35:183–8.
21. Campbell GL, Hills SL, Fischer M, et al. Estimated global incidence of Japanese encephalitis: a systematic review. Bull World Health Organ 2011;89:766–74, 74A–74E.

22. Kaltenbock A, Dubischar-Kastner K, Eder G, et al. Safety and immunogenicity of concomitant vaccination with the cell-culture based Japanese Encephalitis vaccine IC51 and the hepatitis A vaccine HAVRIX1440 in healthy subjects: a single-blind, randomized, controlled Phase 3 study. Vaccine 2009;27:4483–9.
23. Heinz FX, Stiasny K, Holzmann H, et al. Vaccination and tick-borne encephalitis, central Europe. Emerg Infect Dis 2013;19:69–76.
24. Durbin AP, Kirkpatrick BD, Pierce KK, et al. A single dose of any of four different live attenuated tetravalent dengue vaccines is safe and immunogenic in flavivirus-naive adults: a randomized, double-blind clinical trial. J Infect Dis 2013;207:957–65.
25. Schwartz LM, Halloran ME, Durbin AP, et al. The dengue vaccine pipeline: implications for the future of dengue control. Vaccine 2015;33:3293–8.
26. Ouattara A, Laurens MB. Vaccines against malaria. Clin Infect Dis 2015;60:930–6.
27. Lin FY, Ho VA, Khiem HB, et al. The efficacy of a *Salmonella typhi* Vi conjugate vaccine in two-to-five-year-old children. N Engl J Med 2001;344:1263–9.

Promoting Vaccine Confidence

Michael J. Smith, MD, MSCE

KEYWORDS

- Vaccine hesitancy ● Vaccine safety ● Risk communication

KEY POINTS

- Although vaccines are one of the most successful public interventions of all time, some parents remain concerned about vaccine safety.
- Vaccine hesitancy includes a broad spectrum of parental attitudes, beliefs, and behaviors that includes vaccine refusal and intentional vaccine delay.
- Providing parents with reliable evidence-based information about vaccines is an important component of vaccine risk communication.
- Taking a presumptive approach is an effective strategy when discussing vaccines with parents.
- Additional studies identifying the most effective communication strategies for effective vaccine risk communication are needed.

INTRODUCTION

Measles is one of the most contagious infectious diseases known to man. In the prevaccine era in the United States, it was a rite of childhood with millions of cases and several hundred deaths each year. The introduction of the measles, mumps, and rubella (MMR) vaccine, a safe and effective vaccine that confers protection to 97% of recipients after 2 doses, drastically changed the epidemiology of measles, which was declared eliminated from the United States in 2000.

Yet, 2014 saw a significant increase in measles cases in the United States, with 668 cases reported to the Centers for Disease Control and Prevention (CDC), the most in 2 decades. This trend continued during the first 5 months of 2015; as of May 29, 173 individuals from 21 states were reported to have been infected.[1] Of these, 117 (70%) were linked to a single outbreak at a California amusement park.

Disclosure: The author has received research funding as site principal investigator for phase 3 vaccine clinical trials from Novartis and Sanofi. No specific products or off-label indications are discussed in this article.
Division of Pediatric Infectious Diseases, University of Louisville School of Medicine, 571 South Floyd Street, Suite 321, Louisville, KY 40202, USA
E-mail address: mjsmit22@louisville.edu

Infect Dis Clin N Am 29 (2015) 759–769
http://dx.doi.org/10.1016/j.idc.2015.07.004
0891-5520/15/$ – see front matter © 2015 Elsevier Inc. All rights reserved.
id.theclinics.com

Similar to previous outbreaks, most cases occurred in unvaccinated individuals. Some were unvaccinated for medical reasons, either because of age or immune suppression, but many remained unvaccinated because of personal choice. The Disneyland outbreak resulted in significant media coverage and reinvigorated discussions about vaccines in the United States. Countless television, newspaper, and magazine articles called attention to parents who chose to defer or refuse vaccines for their children and squarely blamed them for the outbreak.

Why are parents concerned about vaccines? This article reviews some of the underlying themes and specific examples of vaccine hesitancy in the United States. Strategies for effective vaccine risk communication are also reviewed.

WHAT IS VACCINE HESITANCY ANYWAY?

Vaccine hesitancy is a heterogeneous term that encompasses the entire spectrum of parental vaccine concerns. One definition proposed by a working group from the World Health Organization (WHO) is as follows:

Vaccine hesitancy refers to delay in the acceptance or refusal of vaccination despite availability of vaccination services. Vaccine hesitancy is complex and content specific, varying across time, place and vaccines. It is influenced by factors such as complacency, convenience and confidence.[2]

This working definition captures the key elements of vaccine hesitancy. Perhaps the most important point is that parental vaccine hesitancy is a moving target. It incorporates the concerns of parents who refuse all recommended childhood vaccines as well as those who delay but ultimately accept vaccination. It can refer to a single vaccine or all vaccines, and specific vaccine safety concerns vary from family to family. As a result, any efforts to counter vaccine hesitancy need to be individualized.

The WHO working group attributes vaccine hesitancy to the interaction between complacency, convenience, and confidence in their framework. Complacency refers to the perception that the risks of vaccines outweigh their benefits. Convenience refers to the availability of vaccines, and confidence refers to trust in vaccines themselves, the health care system as a whole, and the policy makers who determine the immunization schedule. Although this framework is new, these concepts are not. This article reviews these concepts and offers talking points that may be used with vaccine-hesitant parents.

HOW COMMON IS VACCINE HESITANCY?

With such a heterogeneous definition, vaccine hesitancy can be difficult to measure. Data from the 2013 National Immunization Survey (NIS) demonstrate that most children in the United States received all recommended vaccines.[3] NIS data do not include reasons for vaccine nonreceipt, so they cannot distinguish intentional parental behavior from missed opportunities or poor access to care. However, it is generally accepted that receipt of no vaccines at all indicates intentional vaccine refusal.[4] Fortunately, less than less than 1% of US children fall into this category. Although there are International Classification of Diseases (ICD)-9 codes for parental vaccine refusal, they are not universally used. Review of immunization records from 157,454 undervaccinated children in the Vaccine Safety Datalink identified almost 1400 unique patterns of immunization.[5] Only 6172 (3.9%) of these records had a specific ICD-9 code consistent with vaccine refusal, suggesting it is not a sensitive metric.

A more reliable measure of vaccine hesitancy may be the prevalence of exemptions to school entry vaccine mandates, which require intentional parental action. It is well documented that the ease of obtaining exemptions in any given state is directly associated with the percentage of exemptions.[6] Nevertheless, exemptions may underestimate vaccine hesitancy as there is significant state to state variation in which vaccines are required and home-schooled children are not included.

Another effective way to assess vaccine hesitancy is to ask parents themselves. A nationally representative survey of parents of young children conducted in 2010 found that 13% of parents used an alternative vaccination schedule (defined as any deviation from the schedule recommended by the Advisory Committee on Immunization Practices).[7] Nearly one-half of the alternative vaccinators (53%) stated that their children did not receive certain vaccines, whereas 17% reported that their children received no vaccines at all. The most commonly *refused* vaccines were related to influenza; 86% refused H1N1 vaccine and 76% refused seasonal vaccine. About 55% reported that they delayed some vaccines until their children were older than the recommended age; the most commonly delayed vaccines were MMR (54%) and varicella (44%). More than 80% of the alternative vaccinators had made more than 1 change to the standard schedule.

Although national estimates of vaccine hesitancy vary based on methodology and specific vaccine concern, it is certain that primary care providers encounter vaccine-hesitant parents in their day to day practice; 93% of physician respondents to a recent national survey reported caring for families who requested spreading out vaccines in a given month.[8] Physicians therefore need to be familiar with the underlying elements of vaccine hesitancy and develop strategies to allay parental concerns.

COMPLACENCY AND VACCINE RISK PERCEPTIONS

Vaccines are one of the greatest public health accomplishments of all time. As a result, they have become a victim of their own success. Because parents do not have personal experience with the devastating effects of vaccine-preventable diseases, they may not view them as important. Furthermore, because vaccines are administered to healthy children to prevent, and not treat, disease, parental threshold for risk is even lower. Any theoretic concern about the safety of childhood vaccines may cause a parent to delay or refuse immunizations. Thus, a key element in effective vaccine risk communication is convincing parents that not vaccinating their children is the greater risk.

The recent measles outbreak in the United States illustrates the importance of vaccination. CDC data through April 2015 demonstrate that most patients with reported measles in the 2015 outbreaks were either unvaccinated (45%) or had unknown vaccination status (38%).[9] Of the US residents who had measles and were unvaccinated, 43% were unvaccinated because of philosophic or religious objections to vaccination. An additional 40% were ineligible because they were too young to receive vaccination or had a medical contraindication. Similar patterns of vaccine receipt have been reported in previous measles outbreaks, and this phenomenon is well supported by the medical literature.

One study published a decade ago demonstrated that children with nonmedical exemptions for MMR were 22 times more likely to contract measles.[10] Those with nonmedical exemptions for pertussis were 5.9 times more likely to develop pertussis as compared with vaccinated controls. In 3 more recent case-control studies that used administrative data from Kaiser Permanente of Colorado, Glanz and colleagues[11] demonstrated that children whose parents had refused one or more immunizations for nonmedical reasons had much higher rates of vaccine-preventable diseases. Children who did not receive pertussis vaccine had a 23-fold increased risk of developing pertussis. The increased risk of disease due to intentional nonreceipt of varicella (8.6) and pneumococcal (6.5) vaccines was smaller but still significant.[12,13] In these 3 studies, vaccine refusal was determined by blinded review of the primary medical record for explicit documentation of parental vaccine refusal. Taken together, these data clearly show that measles, pertussis, and varicella are still prevalent in the United States and that unvaccinated children, specifically those unvaccinated because of parental choice, remain at increased risk. These studies do not, however, prove that vaccines are safe, another key component of risk perception.

CONFIDENCE IN VACCINE SAFETY

Like any other pharmaceutical agent, vaccines may have unintended side effects. Fortunately, most vaccine adverse events are transient and mild. These include fever and injection site reactions such as erythema, warmth, and tenderness. Although they need to be explained to parents, serious vaccine adverse events are extremely uncommon. For instance, a review of 7.5 million vaccine doses from 1991 to 1997 identified only 5 cases of anaphylaxis for an estimated 0.65 cases/million doses administered.[14]

Vaccines are one of the safest and well-studied pharmaceutical agents on the market. Primary care physicians should be familiar with the processes in place to assess vaccine safety in the United States. These include both prelicensure clinical trials and ongoing postlicensure monitoring once a vaccine enters routine use. The main vaccine safety mechanisms in the United States are summarized in **Table 1**. The CDC also sponsors the Clinical Immunization Safety Assessment Project, a network of vaccine safety experts from the CDC's Immunization Safety Office and 7 academic medical centers. This network provides consultative service for individual patients with vaccine adverse events and has generated several vaccine safety research protocols, especially for high-risk populations.

CONFIDENCE IN THE HEALTH CARE SYSTEM

Because vaccine clinical trials are sponsored by the pharmaceutical industry, parents may question their validity. In addition, the fact that many childhood vaccines are mandated as a condition of school entry may raise questions about civil liberties and freedom of choice, a discussion that dates back to the first mandatory smallpox vaccination laws in the United States in 1855. Both of these raise issues of trust with vaccines and the bodies that recommend and enforce them. Fortunately, there is ample evidence that physicians can reassure parents about the safety and necessity of vaccines.

One nationally representative survey found that 82% of parents relied on their child's health care provider for information about vaccinations.[15] In contrast, information from entities such as the CDC (15%) and the American Academy of Pediatrics (21%) was much less commonly used; this underscores the importance of one-on-one communication between a parent and a trusted health care provider. Other studies have confirmed that physicians are the most trustworthy source of immunization information, even for parents who believe vaccines are unsafe and those who request exemptions from childhood vaccines.[16,17] Reassuring information from a health care provider can change the opinions of parents who were initially planning on delaying or refusing a vaccine for their child.[18]

In addition to providing information, physicians can lead by example by vaccinating themselves and their office staff. Health care providers with young children who are up

Table 1
Mechanisms of vaccine safety monitoring in the United States

	Description	Strengths	Limitations
Prelicensure			
Clinical trials	Phase 3 randomized controlled trials with safety and immunogenicity or efficacy end points are required by the US Food and Drug Administration (FDA) before licensure of a new vaccine	Randomization and blinding assure the highest level of epidemiologic evidence	1. Primarily powered to detect efficacy or immunogenicity and common side effects. Rare side effects may not be detected 2. After licensure, it is unethical to randomize children to vaccine receipt and nonreceipt to further evaluate a new safety concern
Postlicensure			
The Vaccine Adverse Events Reporting System	A passive reporting system maintained jointly by the FDA and the CDC that allows anyone (physicians, nurses, parents) who suspects an adverse event to report it	1. Useful for generating hypotheses about vaccine safety that can be further tested using more rigorous epidemiologic methods 2. Inclusive reporting assures generalizability	1. Cannot distinguish temporal association from causation 2. Lack of denominator data preclude ability to calculate incidence of adverse events 3. There may be significant biases in reporting
Vaccine Safety Datalink	Cohort of children from 9 large managed care organizations (MCOs). All medical information, including vaccination status, is entered into medical records as part of routine care. These administrative data can be used to determine associations between vaccines and the outcome of interest	Allows calculation of incidence of adverse events associated with individual vaccines	1. Because it is based on data from MCOs, results may not be generalizable to other populations 2. Because most children in MCOs have adequate immunization rates, cannot compare incidence in vaccinated vs fully unvaccinated children

to date on vaccines can be especially effective communicators with parents who are concerned about vaccines.

ADDRESSING VACCINE HESITANCY

Although primary care physicians are well positioned to convince parents about the safety and necessity of childhood vaccines, the optimal strategies for addressing vaccine hesitancy remain to be elucidated. A recent systematic review identified 30 peer-reviewed studies published between 1990 and 2012 that assessed the impact of various interventions on objective measures of vaccine hesitancy including parental attitudes toward vaccines, intent to vaccinate, and actual vaccine refusal.[19] Of these, 4 focused on introduction of state laws and an additional 3 focused on state and school-level implementation of laws. The remaining 23 studies focused on the use of parent-centered information or education, mostly written educational materials such as pamphlets, brochures, and posters. The effectiveness of these written interventions was mixed; only 8 of 15 educational interventions demonstrated statistically significant increases in parental attitudes toward vaccination and 5 of 10 demonstrated statistically significant increases in parental intention to vaccinate.

Taken together, these studies suggest that providing parents with educational materials may have a positive impact on their attitudes and intentions toward vaccines in at least some cases. Easy access to reliable information about vaccines is a critical component of vaccine risk communication. There are several excellent Web sites designed for parents that address many parental vaccine safety concerns (**Table 2**). However, providers should caution parents to avoid performing their own Google searches, as there is significant misinformation on the Internet, including multiple anti-vaccine Web sites, blogs, and other forms of social media.

It is generally recommended that vaccines be introduced to parents as far in advance of the first well-child visit as possible. Many pediatric offices have developed statements regarding the importance of vaccines that are posted on their Web sites. Additional opportunities include prenatal open houses or during postpartum visits on the maternity ward. Presenting parents with vaccine safety information while they are in the waiting room also provides additional time to reinforce the importance of vaccines.

DELIVERING THE MESSAGE

Although providing parents with information is important, the most critical element in effective vaccine risk communication may be how the message is delivered. Several studies have attempted to address this important question.

Opel and colleagues[20] videotaped interactions between pediatricians and parents during routine office visits, oversampling vaccine-hesitant parents. They were

Table 2
Reliable vaccine Web sites tailored to parents

Organization	Uniform Resource Locator
Children's Hospital of Philadelphia Vaccine Education Center	http://www.vaccine.chop.edu/parents
Immunization Action Coalition	http://www.vaccineinformation.org
Parents of Kids with Infectious Diseases	http://www.pkids.org
Vaccinate Your Baby	http://www.vaccinateyourbaby.com
Voices for Vaccines	http://www.voicesforvaccines.org

particularly interested in how physicians initiated discussions about vaccines. They focused on the use of presumptive approaches, in which the physician assumed parental acceptance of vaccines (eg, "your son needs 3 shots today") as compared with participatory approaches, which allow parents more decision making (eg, "what do you want to do about shots?"). The investigators found that parental resistance to vaccination was less likely when the physicians used a presumptive approach. In contrast, when physicians used participatory approaches vaccine resistance was more common. Just as important as the initial approach was how the physicians responded to parental vaccine resistance. If physicians persisted with their initial recommendation in the face of parental resistance, almost half of the initially resistant parents ultimately accepted vaccination.

A recently published randomized trial assessed the effectiveness of a communication intervention targeted at physicians.[21] The Ask, Acknowledge, Advise strategy was based on risk communication theories and was specifically adapted to vaccine hesitancy. Randomization was performed at the clinic level; 56 clinics in Washington state participated in the study, and 30 were randomized to the intervention. A total of 265 physicians from the 30 clinics were randomized to a 45-minute training session. The primary study outcome was maternal vaccine hesitancy, and the secondary outcome was physicians' confidence in their ability to communicate vaccine safety. The intervention had no statistically significant difference on either of these outcomes. This result may have been because of poor compliance with training; although on-line training was available, only 65% of the physicians randomized to the intervention actually attended an in-person training session.

One of the more interesting findings from this study is physician self-report of confidence in their vaccine risk communication skills. At baseline, 96% of respondents reported confidence in their ability to talk about the benefits of vaccines. However, they were less confident in their ability to provide vaccine information resources (74%), talk about the risks of vaccines (63%), and answer difficult parent questions about vaccines (61%). Although such skills may be learned from years of experience in the office setting, they should be the cornerstone of risk communication training moving forward.

STRATEGIES FOR COMMUNICATING WITH VACCINE-HESITANT PARENTS

Although evidence-based guidelines are lacking, recommendations for discussing vaccine safety with concerned parents have been published (**Box 1**).[22] Most experts agree that interventions need to be targeted to each individual family. Strategies for responding to some of the more common vaccine safety concerns are suggested in the following discussion.

Some parents may be concerned about the number of injections given at a single visit. In a study including 32 pediatric offices, Meyerhoff and Jacobs[23] demonstrated

---

Box 1
Suggested strategies for discussing vaccine safety with parents

Establish honest and respectful dialogue.

Acknowledge that vaccine risks do exist, but balance these against the risks of the disease.

Provide other information sources, such as reputable Internet sites.

Maintain ongoing discussions with vaccine-hesitant families.

that 34% of vaccination visits between 2 and 8 months were associated with deferral of some vaccinations. They found a statistically significant trend between number of vaccine doses due and likelihood of deferral. When 3 or fewer vaccines were due, deferral was only 26%. This value increased to 34% when 4 vaccines were due and 48% when 5 were due. These parents may be reassured by the use of combination vaccines. At the 2-month visit, for example, children receive vaccines against 7 diseases: diphtheria, tetanus, pertussis, polio, pneumococcus, Hib, and rotavirus. One of these is an oral vaccine, and one is a combination vaccine that includes all of the other components except pneumococcal conjugate vaccine. Framing this encounter as "two injections and a drink" may be more effective than "immunization against 7 diseases."

To minimize pain, some parents may request that vaccines be spaced out over several visits. However, there is no difference in stress responses between infants who receive 1 or 2 vaccines.[24] In fact, spacing out vaccines over 2 or 3 visits may actually lead to more stressful stimuli in addition to the inconvenience of extra office visits. Providers should also be familiar with evidence-based strategies that have been shown to reduce immunization pain.[25]

Because most world religions predate vaccines, they are not specifically discussed in religious scriptures. However, certain tenets may affect a family's willingness to vaccinate their children. For instance, cells originally obtained from aborted fetuses are used in certain vaccines such as rubella, as some individuals may object to this. However, these fetuses were not aborted for the purpose of creating these vaccines. Indeed, the Catholic Church has concluded that Catholics may receive these vaccines because they do not contribute to current rates of abortion and are important for the well-being of children and the greater public health. Individuals of Islamic and Jewish faith may have concerns about vaccines containing gelatin as a stabilizer, as it is of porcine origin. Because gelatin is cooked and is not consumed as food, Muslim and Jewish scholars have determined that gelatin-containing vaccines are acceptable.

In addition to the general concerns about vaccines described earlier, parents may have concerns about a specific vaccine or vaccine ingredient. Concise responses to some of the more common parental concerns about vaccines are presented in **Table 3**. The Web sites listed in **Table 4** also contain useful vaccine safety talking points for providers.

PROLOGUE: BACK TO DISNEY

The balance between vaccination and infectious diseases is depicted graphically by the so-called life cycle of an immunization program (**Fig. 1**) Disease incidence begins to decline when a new vaccine is introduced (2). As incidence continues to decrease, adverse vaccine events, both perceived and real, become more prevalent than the disease itself (4). At that point, loss of confidence may develop in a critical proportion of the population (5), and outbreaks may occur (6). Continued decrease in disease incidence with potential disease eradication can only occur after the public is reminded of the severity of infection and people start getting vaccinated again.

Is the 2015 measles outbreak sufficient to reignite confidence in MMR? Only time will tell. A recent pertussis outbreak in Washington did not lead to increases in DTaP immunization.[26] Yet, an outbreak at the happiest place on earth sends a powerful reminder that vaccine-preventable diseases may strike anyone at any time in the United States.

Regardless of the impact of current events on vaccine hesitancy, the aforementioned strategies and talking points should help alleviate some parental concerns.

Table 3
Talking points for common concerns about vaccines

Vaccine Myth	Talking Points
Children should not receive vaccines when they are sick	Presence of moderate or severe acute illness with or without fever is a precaution for vaccine administration; this is not because the vaccine will not work but because the expected side effects of vaccination such as fever or rash might be confused with the natural progression of disease. It is safe to give vaccines to well-appearing children with mild infections such as colds
Natural infection is better than immunization	Although immune protection after natural disease may last a lifetime, natural disease carries greater inherent risk than vaccination. For instance, varicella may result in group A streptococcal superinfection
The MMR vaccine causes autism	In 1998, a small case series published in the *Lancet* claimed an association between MMR and autism. This study only included 12 children, and the results have never been confirmed in larger more rigorous epidemiologic studies. Because of significant ethical concerns in the conduct of this study, it was formally retracted by the journal in 2010
Thimerosal in vaccines causes autism	Multiple epidemiologic studies have found no association between thimerosal and autism. Since the removal of thimerosal from all childhood vaccines, rates of autism in the United States have continued to increase. Today, only certain single-use vials of influenza vaccine still contain thimerosal. Parents who remain concern may request thimerosal-free inactivated vaccine or live-attenuated vaccine
Aluminum in vaccines is unsafe	Aluminum is used as an adjuvant in several vaccines. However, the quantity of aluminum in vaccines is minimal as compared with the aluminum encountered in daily life. Infants are exposed to more aluminum in the form of breast milk and formula than in vaccines
The current immunization schedule is unsafe	The immunization schedule is designed to protect infants against diseases when they are most vulnerable. Delaying vaccines increases the duration of susceptibility against these diseases. Receiving vaccines on time does not increase the likelihood of autism or neurodevelopmental delay
Receiving too many vaccines can overwhelm the immune system	The amount of antigens in childhood vaccines is miniscule compared with those encountered in everyday life; the immune system could theoretically respond to up to 10,000 vaccines at a time.[27] Although the number of vaccines in the childhood schedule has increased, the total antigen burden has decreased, largely because of the discontinuation of smallpox and whole cell pertussis vaccines
Receipt of HPV vaccine leads to promiscuity	A review of medical claims of 1398 adolescent girls found no differences in rates of pregnancy, STI testing, diagnosis, or contraceptive counseling between those who did and did not receive HPV vaccine.[28] Yet, thousands of Americans die each year from vaccine-preventable cancers

Abbreviations: HPV, human papilloma virus; STI, sexually transmitted infection.

Table 4
Reliable vaccine Web sites for health care providers

Organization	Uniform Resource Locator
Centers for Disease Control and Prevention	http://www.cdc.gov/vaccines
American Academy of Pediatrics	http://www.cispimmunize.org
Children's Hospital of Philadelphia Vaccine Education Center	http://www.vaccine.chop.edu

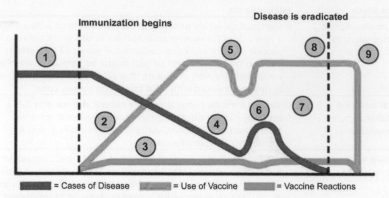

Fig. 1. Life cycle of an immunization program. (*From* Centers for Disease Control. Life cycle of an immunization program. Available at: http://www.cdc.gov/vaccines/vac-gen/life-cycle. htm. *Adapted from* Chen RT, Rastogi SC, Mullen JR, et al. The Vaccine Adverse Event Reporting System (VAERS). Vaccine 1994;12:542–50.)

Further evidence-based recommendations and physician training in vaccine risk communication are needed.

REFERENCES

1. Measles cases and outbreaks. Available at: http://www.cdc.gov/measles/cases-outbreaks.html. Accessed June 2, 2015.
2. MacDonald NE. Vaccine hesitancy: definition, scope and determinants. Vaccine 2015. [Epub ahead of print].
3. Elam-Evans LD, Yankey D, Singleton JA, et al. National, state, and selected local area vaccination coverage among children aged 19-35 months - United States, 2013. MMWR Morb Mortal Wkly Rep 2014;63:741–8.
4. Smith PJ, Chu SY, Barker LE. Children who have received no vaccines: who are they and where do they live? Pediatrics 2004;114:187–95.
5. Louie JK, Schechter R, Honarmand S, et al. Severe pediatric influenza in California, 2003-2005: implications for immunization recommendations. Pediatrics 2006; 117:e610–8.
6. Omer SB, Richards JL, Ward M, et al. Vaccination policies and rates of exemption from immunization, 2005-2011. N Engl J Med 2012;367:1170–1.
7. Dempsey AF, Schaffer S, Singer D, et al. Alternative vaccination schedule preferences among parents of young children. Pediatrics 2011;128:848–56.
8. Kempe A, O'Leary ST, Kennedy A, et al. Physician response to parental requests to spread out the recommended vaccine schedule. Pediatrics 2015;135:666–77.
9. Clemmons NS, Gastanaduy PA, Fiebelkorn AP, et al. Measles - United States, January 4-April 2, 2015. MMWR Morb Mortal Wkly Rep 2015;64:373–6.
10. Feikin DR, Lezotte DC, Hamman RF, et al. Individual and community risks of measles and pertussis associated with personal exemptions to immunization. JAMA 2000;284:3145–50.
11. Glanz JM, McClure DL, Magid DJ, et al. Parental refusal of pertussis vaccination is associated with an increased risk of pertussis infection in children. Pediatrics 2009;123:1446–51.
12. Glanz JM, McClure DL, Magid DJ, et al. Parental refusal of varicella vaccination and the associated risk of varicella infection in children. Arch Pediatr Adolesc Med 2010;164:66–70.

13. Glanz JM, McClure DL, O'Leary ST, et al. Parental decline of pneumococcal vaccination and risk of pneumococcal related disease in children. Vaccine 2011;29:994–9.
14. Bohlke K, Davis RL, Marcy SM, et al. Risk of anaphylaxis after vaccination of children and adolescents. Pediatrics 2003;112:815–20.
15. Kennedy A, Basket M, Sheedy K. Vaccine attitudes, concerns, and information sources reported by parents of young children: results from the 2009 HealthStyles survey. Pediatrics 2011;127(Suppl 1):S92–9.
16. Smith PJ, Kennedy AM, Wooten K, et al. Association between health care providers' influence on parents who have concerns about vaccine safety and vaccination coverage. Pediatrics 2006;118:e1287–92.
17. Salmon DA, Moulton LH, Omer SB, et al. Factors associated with refusal of childhood vaccines among parents of school-aged children: a case-control study. Arch Pediatr Adolesc Med 2005;159:470–6.
18. Gust DA, Darling N, Kennedy A, et al. Parents with doubts about vaccines: which vaccines and reasons why. Pediatrics 2008;122:718–25.
19. Sadaf A, Richards JL, Glanz J, et al. A systematic review of interventions for reducing parental vaccine refusal and vaccine hesitancy. Vaccine 2013;31: 4293–304.
20. Opel DJ, Heritage J, Taylor JA, et al. The architecture of provider-parent vaccine discussions at health supervision visits. Pediatrics 2013;132:1037–46.
21. Henrikson NB, Opel DJ, Grothaus L, et al. Physician communication training and parental vaccine hesitancy: a randomized trial. Pediatrics 2015;136(1):70–9.
22. Healy CM, Pickering LK. How to communicate with vaccine-hesitant parents. Pediatrics 2011;127(Suppl 1):S127–33.
23. Meyerhoff AS, Jacobs RJ. Do too many shots due lead to missed vaccination opportunities? Does it matter? Prev Med 2005;41:540–4.
24. Ramsay DS, Lewis M. Developmental change in infant cortisol and behavioral response to inoculation. Child Dev 1994;65:1491–502.
25. Schechter NL, Zempsky WT, Cohen LL, et al. Pain reduction during pediatric immunizations: evidence-based review and recommendations. Pediatrics 2007; 119:e1184–98.
26. Wolf ER, Opel D, DeHart MP, et al. Impact of a pertussis epidemic on infant vaccination in Washington state. Pediatrics 2014;134:456–64.
27. Offit PA, Quarles J, Gerber MA, et al. Addressing parents' concerns: do multiple vaccines overwhelm or weaken the infant's immune system? Pediatrics 2002;109: 124–9.
28. Bednarczyk RA, Davis R, Ault K, et al. Sexual activity-related outcomes after human papillomavirus vaccination of 11- to 12-year-olds. Pediatrics 2012;130: 798–805.

Index

Note: Page numbers of article titles are in **boldface** type.

Infect Dis Clin N Am 29 (2015) 771–778
http://dx.doi.org/10.1016/S0891-5520(15)00109-9
0891-5520/15/$ – see front matter © 2015 Elsevier Inc. All rights reserved.

id.theclinics.com

United States Postal Service

Statement of Ownership, Management, and Circulation
(All Periodicals Publications Except Requester Publications)

1. Publication Title	2. Publication Number							3. Filing Date
Infectious Disease Clinics of North America	0	0	1	-	5	5	6	9/18/15

4. Issue Frequency	5. Number of Issues Published Annually	6. Annual Subscription Price
Mar, Jun, Sep, Dec	4	$295.00

7. Complete Mailing Address of Known Office of Publication *(Not printer)* *(Street, city, county, state, and ZIP+4®)*

Elsevier Inc.
360 Park Avenue South
New York, NY 10010-1710

Contact Person
Stephen R. Bushing
Telephone *(Include area code)*
215-239-3688

8. Complete Mailing Address of Headquarters or General Business Office of Publisher *(Not printer)*

Elsevier Inc., 360 Park Avenue South, New York, NY 10010-1710

9. Full Names and Complete Mailing Addresses of Publisher, Editor, and Managing Editor *(Do not leave blank)*

Publisher *(Name and complete mailing address)*

Linda Belfus, Elsevier Inc., 1600 John F. Kennedy Blvd., Suite 1800, Philadelphia, PA 19103

Editor *(Name and complete mailing address)*

Kerry Holland, Elsevier Inc., 1600 John F. Kennedy Blvd., Suite 1800, Philadelphia, PA 19103-2899

Managing Editor *(Name and complete mailing address)*

Adrianne Brigido, Elsevier Inc., 1600 John F. Kennedy Blvd., Suite 1800, Philadelphia, PA 19103-2899

10. Owner *(Do not leave blank. If the publication is owned by a corporation, give the name and address of the corporation immediately followed by the names and addresses of all stockholders owning or holding 1 percent or more of the total amount of stock. If not owned by a corporation, give the names and addresses of the individual owners. If owned by a partnership or other unincorporated firm, give its name and address as well as those of each individual owner. If the publication is published by a nonprofit organization, give its name and address.)*

Full Name	Complete Mailing Address
Wholly owned subsidiary of	1600 John F. Kennedy Blvd, Ste. 1800
Reed/Elsevier, US holdings	Philadelphia, PA 19103-2899

11. Known Bondholders, Mortgagees, and Other Security Holders Owning or Holding 1 Percent or More of Total Amount of Bonds, Mortgages, or Other Securities. If none, check box ☑ None

Full Name	Complete Mailing Address
N/A	

12. Tax Status *(For completion by nonprofit organizations authorized to mail at nonprofit rates) (Check one)*
The purpose, function, and nonprofit status of this organization and the exempt status for federal income tax purposes:
☐ Has Not Changed During Preceding 12 Months
☐ Has Changed During Preceding 12 Months *(Publisher must submit explanation of change with this statement)*

13. Publication Title	14. Issue Date for Circulation Data Below
Infectious Disease Clinics of North America	September 2015

15. Extent and Nature of Circulation		Average No. Copies Each Issue During Preceding 12 Months	No. Copies of Single Issue Published Nearest to Filing Date
a. Total Number of Copies *(Net press run)*		681	585
b. Legitimate Paid and/or Requested Distribution (By Mail and Outside the Mail)	(1) Mailed Outside-County Paid/Requested Mail Subscriptions stated on PS Form 3541. *(Include paid distribution above nominal rate, advertiser's proof copies and exchange copies)*	370	302
	(2) Mailed In-County Paid/Requested Mail Subscriptions stated on PS Form 3541. *(Include paid distribution above nominal rate, advertiser's proof copies and exchange copies)*		
	(3) Paid Distribution Outside the Mails Including Sales Through Dealers And Carriers, Street Vendors, Counter Sales, and Other Paid Distribution Outside USPS®	114	125
	(4) Paid Distribution by Other Classes of Mail Through the USPS (e.g. First-Class Mail®)		
c. Total Paid and or Requested Circulation *(Sum of 15b (1), (2), (3), and (4))* ▲		484	427
d. Free or Nominal Rate Distribution (By Mail and Outside the Mail)	(1) Free or Nominal Rate Outside-County Copies included on PS Form 3541	19	14
	(2) Free or Nominal Rate In-County Copies included on PS Form 3541		
	(3) Free or Nominal Rate Copies mailed at Other classes Through the USPS (e.g. First-Class Mail®)		
	(4) Free or Nominal Rate Distribution Outside the Mail *(Carriers or Other means)*		
e. Total Nonrequested Distribution *(Sum of 15d (1), (2), (3) and (4))*		19	14
f. Total Distribution *(Sum of 15c and 15e)* ▲		503	441
g. Copies not Distributed *(See instructions to publishers #4 (page #3))* ▲		178	144
h. Total *(Sum of 15f and g)*		681	585
i. Percent Paid and/or Requested Circulation *(15c divided by 15f times 100)* ▲		96.22%	96.83%

* If you are claiming electronic copies go to line 16 on page 3. If you are not claiming Electronic copies, skip to line 17 on page 3.

16. Electronic Copy Circulation	Average No. Copies Each Issue During Preceding 12 Months	No. Copies of Single Issue Published Nearest to Filing Date
a. Paid Electronic Copies		
b. Total paid Print Copies (Line 15c) + Paid Electronic copies (Line 16a)		
c. Total Print Distribution (Line 15f) + Paid Electronic copies (Line 16a)		
d. Percent Paid (Both Print & Electronic copies) (16b divided by 16c X 100)		

☐ I certify that 50% of all my distributed copies *(electronic and print) are paid above a nominal price*

17. Publication of Statement of Ownership
☑ If the publication is a general publication, publication of this statement is required. Will be printed in the **December 2015** issue of this publication.

18. Signature and Title of Editor, Publisher, Business Manager, or Owner	Date
Stephen R. Bushing	September 18, 2015
Stephen R. Bushing – Inventory Distribution Coordinator	

I certify that all information furnished on this form is true and complete. I understand that anyone who furnishes false or misleading information on this form or who omits material or information requested on the form may be subject to criminal sanctions (including fines and imprisonment) and/or civil sanctions (including civil penalties).

PS Form **3526**, July 2014 (Page 3 of 3)

PS Form **3526**, July 2014 (Page 1 of 3 (Instructions Page 3)) PSN 7530-01-000-9931 **PRIVACY NOTICE:** See our Privacy policy in www.usps.com

Moving?

Make sure your subscription moves with you!

To notify us of your new address, find your **Clinics Account Number** (located on your mailing label above your name), and contact customer service at:

Email: journalscustomerservice-usa@elsevier.com

800-654-2452 (subscribers in the U.S. & Canada)
314-447-8871 (subscribers outside of the U.S. & Canada)

Fax number: 314-447-8029

Elsevier Health Sciences Division
Subscription Customer Service
3251 Riverport Lane
Maryland Heights, MO 63043

*To ensure uninterrupted delivery of your subscription,
please notify us at least 4 weeks in advance of move.

Printed and bound by CPI Group (UK) Ltd, Croydon, CR0 4YY

03/10/2024

01040494-0019